THE AUTHOR has had unusual facilities for studying this entire subject practically as well as scientifically, and has here given the results not only of his own experience, but also those of many skillful experts in veterinary practice. This book is the result of many years' experience with farm horses as well as those used for all other purposes, and is an up-to-date and thoroughly practical treatise on the diseases of the horse. The writer emphasizes the early recognition, the causes and prevention of common diseases, and gives brief and popular advice on the nature and treatment of disease, the common ailments, and the care and management of horses when sick.

The principal purpose of this book is to enable those who, for pleasure or business, own or use a horse, to perform a helpful service and to help in preventing as many diseases as possible, that might otherwise affect his horses.

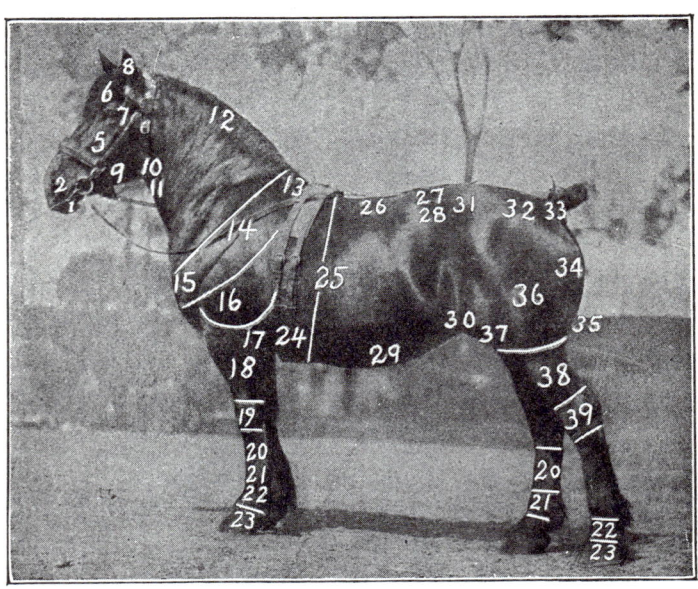

The Points of The Horse: 1, chin; 2, nostril; 4, nose; 5, face; 6, forehead; 7, eye; 8, ear; 9, lower jaw; 10, throat-latch; 11, windpipe; 12, crest; 13, withers; 14, shoulder; 15, joint shoulder; 16, arm; 17, elbow; 18, forearm; 19, knee; 20, cannon; 21, fetlock joint; 22, pastern; 23, hoof; 24, foreflank; 25, hearth girth; 26, back; 27, loin; 28, coupling; 29, belly; 30, hindflank; 31, hip; 32, croup; 33, tail; 34, buttocks; 35, quarters; 38, gaskin; 39, hock.

Treating Common Diseases of Your Horse

by

GEORGE H. CONN, B.S.A.H., D.V.M.

ILLUSTRATED

1974 EDITION

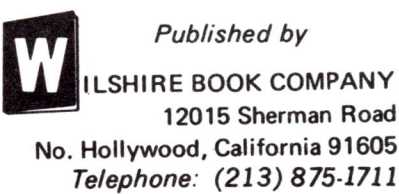

Published by
Wilshire Book Company
12015 Sherman Road
No. Hollywood, California 91605
Telephone: (213) 875-1711

> Printed by
> HAL LEIGHTON PRINTING CO.
> P. O. Box 1231
> Beverly Hills, California 90213
> Telephone: (213) 346-8500

COPYRIGHT, 1942, BY
ORANGE JUDD PUBLISHING COMPANY, INC.

PRINTED IN THE UNITED STATES OF AMERICA

This book or any part thereof may not be reproduced without permission of the publishers, except by a reviewer who wishes to quote brief passages in connection with a review for inclusion in a magazine or a newspaper.

Copyright under the Articles of the Copyright Convention
of the Pan American Republics and the
United States August 11, 1910
ISBN 0-87980-255-3

TABLE OF CONTENTS

CHAPTER		PAGE
I.	THE STABLE AND ITS EQUIPMENT	15
II.	SECURING THE HORSE IN THE STABLE	29
III.	STABLE CLOTHING AND BEDDING FOR THE HORSE	37
IV.	STABLE TRICKS AND VICES OF THE HORSE	47
V.	GROOMING THE HORSE	57
VI.	HOW TO HANDLE THE HORSE	69
VII.	CLIPPING THE HORSE	79
VIII.	SOME CAUSES OF DISEASE IN THE HORSE	86
IX.	HOW TO TELL THE SICK HORSE	92
X.	THE VALUE OF EXERCISE AND CONDITION IN PREVENTING DISEASE	96
XI.	HOW TO GIVE MEDICINES TO THE HORSE	103
XII.	GENERAL CARE OF THE SICK HORSE	110
XIII.	COLIC OR INDIGESTION	117
XIV.	DISEASES OF THE BREATHING SYSTEM	127
XV.	DISEASES OF THE FEET AND LEGS	135
XVI.	CONTAGIOUS DISEASES	151
XVII.	MISCELLANEOUS DISEASES	167
XVIII.	DISEASES OF YOUNG FOALS	176

LIST OF ILLUSTRATIONS

	PAGE
A Practical Horse Barn with Some Box Stalls	16
A Horse Barn with Only Tie Stalls	19
A Horse Barn with Nothing but Box Stalls	21
A Good Type Percheron Mare	30
Give Medicine to Horse in a Capsule	31
Draft Mares and Colts	33
Mares and Foals at Pasture	35
Horse Lame in Front Foot	38
Horse with Jack (Spavin)	97
How to Fit a Horse's Collar	48
The Horse Collar Should Be Long Enough	51
A Poultice for a Sore Throat	55
A Horse with a Ewe Neck (Faulty Conformation)	58
The Teeth of a Young Horse	60
The Teeth of an Old Horse	64
Breaking a Colt to Lead	69
A War Bridle	71
A War (or Pulley) Bridle	73
A Horse or Breeding Hopple	74
Casting or Throwing Harness	76
Horse with Bog Spavin	80
Horse with Curb	83

LIST OF ILLUSTRATIONS

	PAGE
Where to Count the Horse's Pulse	94
Horse with Set Hock	128
Horse with Wind Gall (or Wind Puff)	101
Horse with Sidebone	131
Percheron Mare with Colt	105
How to Drenche a Horse	107
Horse That Is Stifled	111
Hind Leg Too Straight	113
Horse with Colic	119
Horse with Capped Hock	41
Horse with Shoe Boil	99
Too Long in Gaskin	136
Horse with Ringbones	139
Horse That Is Cock-Ankled	142
Foundered Foot	146
Faulty Conformation of the Front Legs	153
Horse Badly Infested with Worms	156
Horse After Being Wormed	169
Horse with Lock Jaw	174
Fistula of the Withers	177
Colt with Navel Rupture	181

PREFACE TO
SOME COMMON DISEASES OF HORSES

My early life was spent on the farm when horses were the principal and almost the only farm power available—also when the horse was the principal source of transportation. In fact, during the first years of my practice horses were used exclusively by me to serve my clients.

My veterinary experience with horses has extended for a period of more than 25 years. This experience has consisted of contact and personal experiences with farm horses, drayage horses, trotters and pacers, saddle horses, show horses and army horses. During the World War I, I assisted in the purchase of 50,000 head of army horses and mules and the care of 100,000 more. At some remounts we had as many as 12,000 head.

The information given in this book is the result of an extensive and wide experience with the horse in health and disease. It is given for the principal purpose of helping the horse owner to provide better care for his charges and to be of greater assistance to his veterinarian through the knowledge of his inability to render adequate veterinary service to his horses, which only a veterinarian can do effectively.

There are certain minor conditions that do not often require a veterinarian's attention, and in other cases a veterinarian is not always available; in such cases the horse owner will find much information in this book that will be helpful to him.

The principal purpose of this book is to enable the owner to perform a more helpful service to his horses and to help in preventing as far as practical as many diseases as possible, that might otherwise affect his horses.

GEORGE H. CONN

Freeport, Ill.

SOME COMMON DISEASES
OF THE HORSE

CHAPTER I

THE STABLE AND ITS EQUIPMENT

It is not the intention of the author to attempt to state just how the barn should be built, but it is our aim to point out those desirable features of a practical utility stable. It is necessary if one would obtain the greatest service from his horses to provide a shelter for them. The kind of a barn that is necessary is largely determined by the climatic conditions, and may be influenced some by the amount of work the animal has to perform. A stable that would be ideal for one owner might not do for another man at all, due to the local conditions that are present. However, there are certain features that should be found in most barns, and in this discussion we will consider them as to their health, permanence, and convenience. Each man in planning a stable can do so, approximating this as near as local conditions will indicate.

Location of the Stable

To our mind this is one of the most important features concerning the erection of a stable. It is important for several reasons; it may save labor in caring for the animals; lessens the dangers of the acquiring of disease; adds to the appearance of the home-

16 SOME COMMON DISEASES OF THE HORSE

stead and makes the best use of the natural elements, the sunlight and the air.

The stable should always be located on ground that has as much natural drainage as possible. This

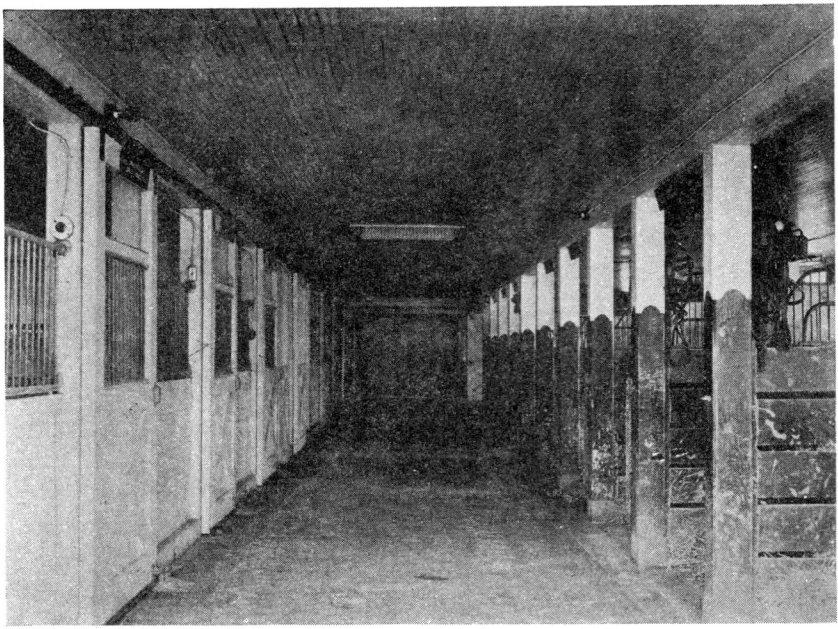

This shows a practical horse barn for the horse owner who wants to raise some colts each year. Box stalls are necessary for best results in raising colts. *Courtesy James Mfg. Co., Ft. Atkinson, Wis.*

will place the barn as far above the water line as possible. A stable located in a low wet spot will be damp and unhealthy. It should be located so as to provide pure air and an abundance of sunlight. The surrounding buildings and the prevailing winds should

THE STABLE AND ITS EQUIPMENT

always be taken into consideration. If possible, it is best to place the stable with the house between the stable and the prevailing winds, or odors from the barn may become very obnoxious at various times. In most sections the cold winds usually come from the north and west, and for this reason horses should if possible be stabled on the south or the east side of the building. If they are placed on the south side they will receive a greater amount of sunlight than from any other location. This not only assists in keeping the animals healthy but adds to the cheerfulness of the surroundings.

A hard clay, limestone or gravelly soil is much better for the location of a stable than black, mucky, peaty soil. Where the latter is used it is usually necessary to subdrain the soil thoroughly. In these soils it requires much more care in the building of the foundation and the floor.

In some sections of the country bank barns are very common. They are objectionable for this reason, that they can very rarely be ventilated properly, are usually dark, and quite often cold and damp. It is a fact that in many large stables of this kind many horses suffer from periodic ophthalmia or moon-blindness, and that they often go blind.

Importance of Ventilation

Ventilation of the stable is the act of keeping the air of the building approximately pure, to draw out the excessive moisture, to retain enough heat in the stable to keep the animals comfortable while it is closed and filled with stock. It requires a certain kind of structure in many climates to carry out this ventilation properly, but these facts can be supplied in detail by a ventilating company.

According to W. B. Clarkson of the King Ventilating Company, in a stable not ventilated a 1,400 pound horse requires 1,500 cubic feet of air space; in the stable that is properly ventilated this same horse can be maintained very satisfactorily in 730 cubic feet of air space. This is a great saving in space; more than enough to provide for the ventilation if it had no other good features. It removes the moisture from the stable that is given off by the animals during respiration; this is a very valuable feature as we know that animals do not often suffer from the cold in a stable in which the air is dry. According to the late Prof. F. H. King, the stable at no time should contain more than three and three-tenths per cent of air that has been once breathed, and that to keep the breathed air down to this per cent it must enter and leave the stable at the rate of 71.6 cubic feet per minute; this is based upon a horse weighing 1,400 pounds.

It is impractical if not impossible to think of securing proper ventilation for the barn, without installing the proper devices for securing the desired results. The doors and windows through which the ventilation must all take place in the barn that has

THE STABLE AND ITS EQUIPMENT 19

no ventilating system, must be permanent and this makes it impossible to secure the desired results due to the shifting of the direction of the wind. If it were possible to always have the air currents coming

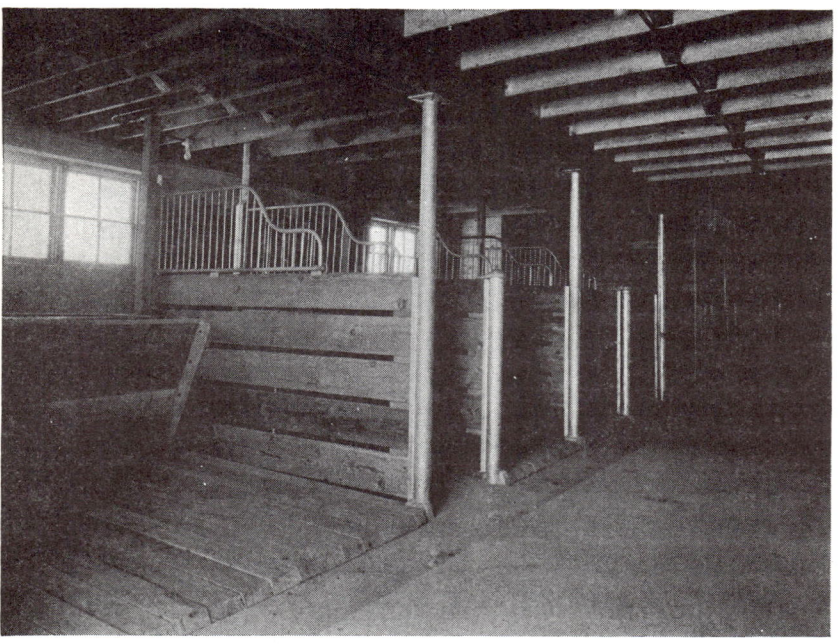

This barn is of strong, rugged construction and should provide good housing for work horses. *Courtesy James Mfg. Co., Ft. Atkinson, Wis.*

from the same direction, and with about the same velocity, it might then be possible to ventilate the stable fairly successfully by using the windows and doors.

In using the doors and windows for ventilating

purposes drafts are very apt to result, and during rain and snow storms, they permit much moisture gaining access to the stable. From our experience and that of many men of good judgment, we can hardly understand why anyone should build a stable for animals without installing a thorough and efficient ventilating system. They practically all are built upon the same principle and there is very little preference between them as far as we know. However, the ones made from galvanized iron or metal would no doubt be the cheapest and most satisfactory in the long run. In building a stable it would be advisable to submit plans to the engineers of some large ventilating company, who could advise you upon the ventilation of the proposed structure.

Materials Used

In times past, most stables were built entirely of wood. The growing scarcity of wood and its correspondingly high price makes it necessary that we use other building materials such as brick and concrete.

These two substances make very good stable walls when properly constructed, but when care is not used they are very unsatisfactory due to the dampness.

Concrete is rapidly growing in favor as a building material, but where animal life is to be housed in the structure the greatest of care must be used to secure the best results. Before building a stable of

THE STABLE AND ITS EQUIPMENT

either concrete or blocks, it would be advisable to interview several owners of this kind of stable and secure the results of their experience.

The Floor

Without a doubt the concrete floor is the most popular of any floor that has ever been used in the stable. There are some objections to it, however, but most of them can be overcome fairly satisfac-

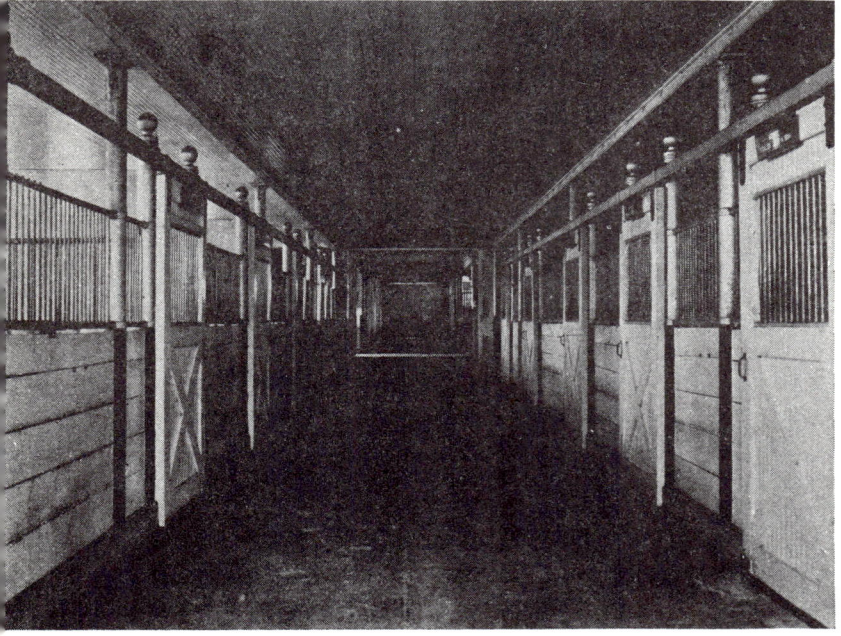

This barn has all box stalls and should be very satisfactory for a breeding or sale barn. Horses are more easily kept clean and comfortable in box stalls. *Courtesy James Mfg. Co., Ft. Atkinson, Wis.*

torily. It may be damp if the stable is located where the water level is high, but this can be overcome by sub-draining, the use of a layer of cinders or crushed stone under the floor to facilitate drainage and by a layer of flat tile below the floor or within the floor; also by special construction of the floor. The concrete floor is cold, but this can be taken care of by a supply of bedding in the stall. It is also smooth, and horses must be handled very carefully to prevent injury from slipping; this can be prevented largely by roughing the surface of the floor.

It also has many advantages; it is permanent; easily cleaned; sanitary; does not have any space beneath for the circulation of cold air, and for harboring rats and mice; does not have any cracks for the accumulation of dirt, disease germs and filth; will not absorb the liquid manure and the urine, thus preventing bad odors. The floor should slope two inches in ten feet to drain off the urine properly.

The Windows

In our judgment most stable windows are placed much too low; they should not be for the animal to use for looking out, but for the admission of sunlight. When they are too low and are left open the air produces a draft that hits the animal squarely; when placed higher it will pass above them. Windows should be placed eight feet from the floor, should be hinged at the bottom and should open inward; during cold windy days those windows on the leeward side may be kept open, and on calm days those on both sides. There should be one window for each horse and should provide a space of at least four square feet. It should contain glasses of small dimensions rather than one large glass, as they are not so easily broken; usually two or four panes make the best size for small windows. The glass can be protected by slats of wood or metal or by wire screen.

The Stalls

The ideal stall for the most comfort of the horse is the box stall, where space and the number of horses will permit, and the expense is not too great, this type of stall is to be recommended. It should be about 10 x 12 feet for use as a foaling stall.

The tie stalls should be roomy to provide comfort for the horse; they should be 11 feet from wall to heel posts, and five feet six inches from center to center. For cribbers it might be well to make the stall six feet wide. It requires about 18 feet of space for one row of stalls and about 30 feet for the two rows. The stalls should face toward the walls.

Since lumber of good quality is very high in price it is advisable to use the steel fixtures that several manufacturers are putting upon the market; they have these advantages: are sanitary, finely appearing, durable, strong, require little attention when properly installed and can be easily kept clean. No doubt when the length of time they will last is considered they are cheaper than wood by quite a large per cent, comparing the original cost of both.

The Manger

With the large amounts of saliva that are drivelled into the manger or feed box, for sanitary reasons the iron manger is the only one that is to be recommended. It should be wide and shallow and not short and deep; this prevents a great waste of grain. It should be easily cleaned. A manger should have perfectly smooth surfaces and have rounding corners. A rim projecting inward from the top usually prevents the wasting of feed, but it should be so constructed that dirt and spoiled feed will not accumulate. It should be placed about $3\frac{1}{2}$ feet from the floor.

The Hay Racks

They should be on a level with the manger; they should be fairly deep and wide and long. Hay racks that are placed above the horse's head may be the means of the animal getting dirt or chaff in the eyes, and besides much hay is wasted by the animals pulling it down to be eaten; some of the hay will fall to the floor and it will be soiled and trampled. With usual high prices it would require only a small quantity of feeds being wasted to pay for the best of hay racks. A loose hay rack is to be discouraged due to the waste. Hay racks should be thoroughly cleaned and disinfected so that they will not permit of a large collection of dirt and trash.

Stable Doors

They should be at least eight feet high and four feet wide. With a narrow low door the nervous horse is not only apt to injure himself by striking the side of the door, but he is also liable to injure the attendant by crowding when going through the door. Many a good horse has been injured by a door that was too narrow. We are of the opinion that the two section door is the one that is in the most common use; by making the door in two sections, the lower part can be closed while the upper part is left open. Should be hung on strong T hinges. If made in two sections the lower section should be of sufficient height that an animal would not attempt to jump over it.

If the door is made in one section only it can best be placed upon a track with rollers. Such a door does not work so well upon hinges as it does by rolling on a track.

Latches, Catches and Fasteners

They should all be considered as to practicability, adaptability, durability, construction, ease of operating and location.

They should all be so placed that there will be no

sharp projections upon which the horse may become injured. Such injuries may be of very little concern at times, but at other times they may produce a very serious injury that may endanger the animal's life, or greatly affect his market value.

Stable Drainage

Under no circumstance is it advisable to drain a stall from the center; by that we mean the putting of the drain in the center of the stall; this is the source of ammonia vapors and obnoxious odors from the urine, which are detrimental to the best health of the animal; and to say the least is very unsanitary. By sloping the stall two inches in every ten feet, the urine can be drained to the rear of the stall, where a shallow gutter can be made; if the stable is less than 20 feet this gutter can slope to either end of the stable and empty into a drain. If the stable is more than 20 feet, and up to 40 feet, it will be best to make the slope both ways from the center of the stable, and have a drain at both ends of the stable. If the barn is long and it is desired to have the drain in the stable, it will be best to have the slope from each end of the stable, toward the center. If the drain is placed in the stable, a suitable trap should be placed to prevent the return of any sewer gas or obnoxious odors. There is also difficulty in getting at the drains to unstop them. When they are placed in the stable they frequently become clogged from small particles of bedding, and dust and dirt that wash into them.

Everything considered, draining the urine and liquid manure to the outside of the stable to a suitable catch-basin, will give the best results and save a lot of expense in getting at the one in the stable when it clogs up, and will in the end prove much more satisfactory.

The Litter Carrier

During the past few years the price of farm labor has made some wonderful increases; it is also difficult to keep farm labor, due many times to the lack of labor saving devices. There was a time when the farm laborer expected to perform most of his work by "main strength and awkwardness" as the old saying goes, but they have not been slow to note the improved labor saving devices, consequently they are more easily secured and kept where the farmer has an up-to-date equipment.

The litter carrier can be installed in practically any stable and it is an exceedingly convenient means of handling the manure and litter from the stable. It will save enough in labor in the course of a few months to pay for it. It consists of a large metal receptacle for holding the litter, which is suspended by two chains, which are fastened to a carrier that travels on a track that is suspended from the sills of the ceiling. This track can be placed at any place in the barn and the height of the carrier can be adjusted.

The Feed Carrier

It is a large box for carrying the feed to the horses. It can be used upon the same track as the litter carrier. Where there is a large number of animals to be fed, it will reduce the labor cost very materially. Aside from this item they are very convenient.

CHAPTER II

SECURING THE HORSE IN THE STABLE

There are several methods by which horses are secured in the stable, but each has its advantages and disadvantages. For the reason that so few practical horsemen can give an intelligent description of a practical method, and the reasons for such methods, it was thought best to give it some attention here. Not all horsemen are partial to the same method of securing the horse, but the method to use will depend largely upon the nature of the horse and the preference of the attendant.

The aims that are sought in securing the horse are to secure firmly so that he cannot get loose, to prevent his becoming injured in the fastenings and to make him as comfortable as possible and to provide as much freedom of movement as is possible without danger of becoming injured.

In the U.S. we speak of all fittings for the head as a halter. In England, a halter is made of rope and consists of a head stall and side checks, nose band, back rope and tie. The leather halter, as we term it, is known as a head collar and has a head stall, brow band, throat lash, nose band, back strap and tie strap; they are known as head collars. However, halters with brow bands are not used to any extent upon work horses in the U.S. Horses are also secured by placing a broad strap about the neck, upon which a ring is placed; this is most often used in halter pullers.

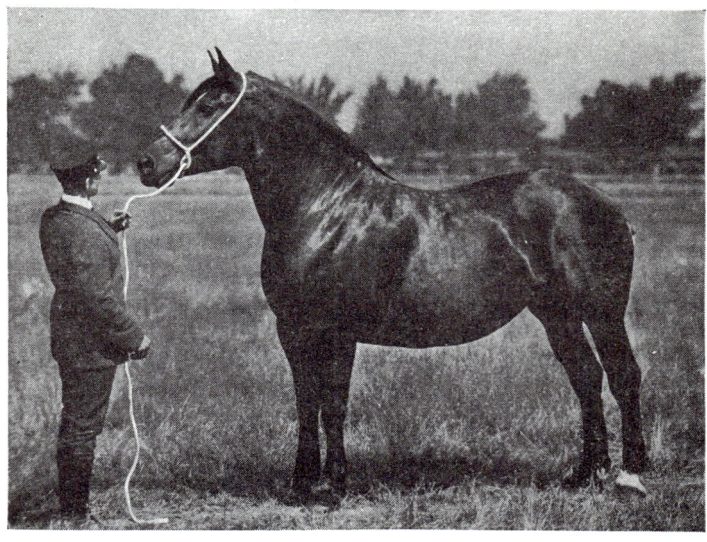

This good percheron mare can do her part of the farm work and raise a valuable colt each year. Costs no more to feed and care for a good one than it does a cheap one, but the income should be much greater.
Courtesy U.S. Dept. of Agriculture.

Fitting the Halter

There are several difficulties that must be watched for in fitting the halter with a brow band; if the brow band is too short it will pull the head stall too close against the horses' ears and cut them; it may

SECURING THE HORSE IN THE STABLE

also be the means of making the cheek bones sore from pulling the cheek pieces forward against them. This often causes the animal to rub the back of its head, and in this way the halter is often removed and many a horse becomes a confirmed halter puller.

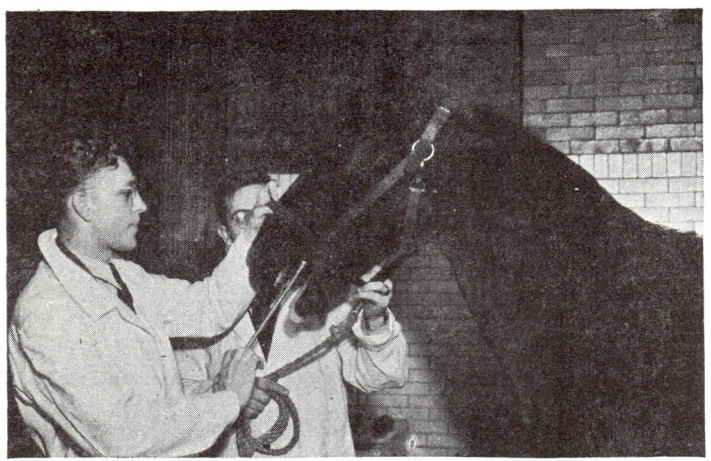

Giving a capsule or bolus to a horse with a balling gun. *Courtesy Prof. R. S. Hudson, Michigan State College.*

In a halter of this kind the brow band should be just long enough that the cheek pieces do not make the cheek bones sore, nor the head stall cut the base of the ears. The throat latch must be buckled just tight enough that it does not interfere with the animal's swallowings; the throat latch may be sewed on the side pieces or cheeks of the halter or it may be made of a single strap passing through the loops of the brow band and over the top of the head. The cheeks should extend to just above the animal's mouth; about 2½ to 3 inches is about the proper distance. The nose band should be wide and strong and just long enough that the checks form a straight line from the poll. The back strap should be long enough to permit the movements of the animal's jaws while eating and during yawning.

The tie strap should be just of sufficient length to reach from the back strap of the halter to the floor, when the horse is standing naturally. If the animal is fastened by tying, the length of the strap from the halter to the manger where it is tied should be sufficient length to reach from the manger to the floor; this will permit the animal to lie down with comfort.

Fastening to Manger

It is a practice by some to use a chain and a log; the objection to the chain is the noise they make; the advantage is their strength and durability. A log is simply a weight of iron or wood, and is for the purpose of drawing the chain taut at all times. When fastening by this method the log must be heavy enough to draw the chain through the hole in the manger at all times, otherwise a large loop of chain may be the means of the animal injuring itself by becoming caught in it. The hole in the manger must be large enough that the chain will not be easily caught, and the chain is passed through from the outside and the log is directly behind the manger,

SECURING THE HORSE IN THE STABLE 33

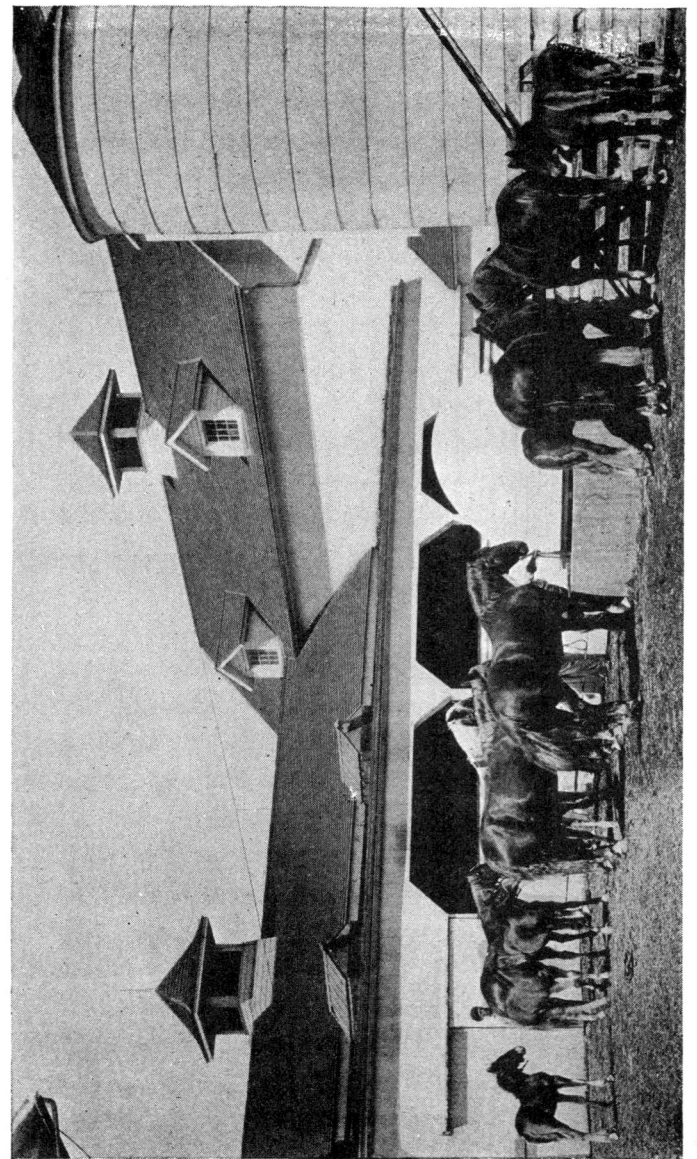

These draft mares and colts are valuable farm property and will bring in a good yearly income. *Courtesy U.S. Dept. of Agriculture.*

34 SOME COMMON DISEASES OF THE HORSE

just in front of the animal's feet. Straps and rope ties do not work so well with a log as they are quite apt to become fastened or twisted in passing through the hole in the manger. The chain must be long enough that the log can lie on the floor when the animal is standing naturally, and yet be taut.

If a chain is to be used, the following method will no doubt be the best. Take a heavy iron rod and fasten to the edge of the manger and fasten the other end to the floor just at the bottom of the manger. This rod is on the outside of the manger and close enough to the manger that the horse cannot catch a shoe or its foot; upon this rod is welded a heavy iron ring that will slide up and down. A piece of chain 2½ feet long is fastened to this ring and the other end to the halter. It is a very satisfactory method of fastening.

Slipping the Halter

As mentioned above this trick is apt to be learned if the horse wears a halter with a brow band, especially if it makes the ears and head sore. The horse either rubs its head under the edge of the manger or gets the tie over the top of the head, and slips it off by pulling back. In such cases the brow band should be removed and the throat latch tightened so that the head stall will rest farther back on the poll. The manger may be boarded up from the edge to the floor, but no doubt the best way is to use a broad

SECURING THE HORSE IN THE STABLE

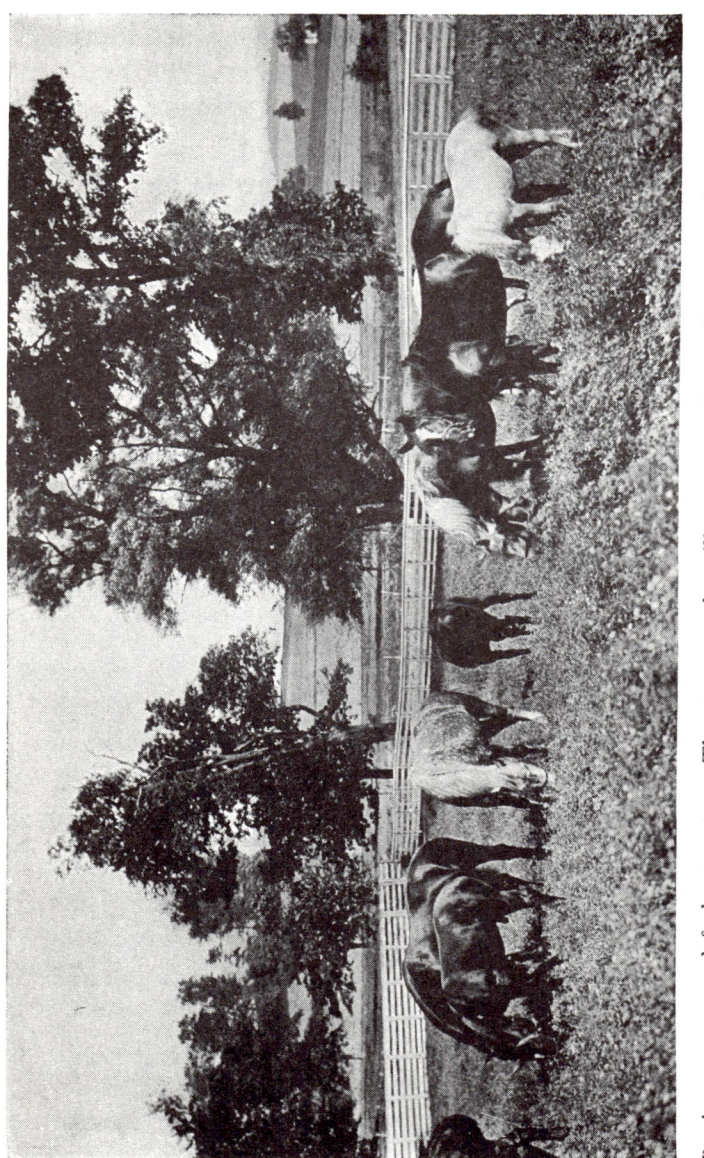

Percheron mares and foals at pasture. These young colts will soon grow into real money and will add to the farmer's income. *Courtesy of U.S. Dept. of Agriculture.*

stout strap about the neck, just tight enough that the animal can swallow without any discomfort.

Cross-Tying

At times it may be necessary to tie an animal to one or either side of a stall or to keep it in a special position; occasionally an animal is tied for the purpose of having it lie on one particular side. This can be accomplished by using two ties one in either ring of the side cheeks. If it is desired that the animal lie on the left side while lying down shorten the right tie and lengthen the left one; if it is desired that the horse lie on the right side reverse this procedure.

CHAPTER III

STABLE CLOTHING AND BEDDING FOR THE HORSE

The Need of Clothing

During the winter months blankets are usually used, when horses have been clipped. There is not much doubt but that they are of much value, inasmuch as a lot of feed may be saved, or at least a lot of energy that goes to produce heat will be saved by the use of a blanket. Hardly anyone would dispute this latter fact. It also adds to the appearance of the animal by producing a better coat of hair, and it materially adds to the comfort of the animal. While we have determined that the animal really does not need a blanket to keep in good health, yet the saving in feed, the improvement in the appearance, and the comfort it gives the animal, are reasons enough to influence the common use of the blanket upon horses during the winter months.

The Type of Blanket

The blanket first of all must be of material that will be warm, that is strong and will not be easily torn, and material that can be kept reasonably clean. Two common materials for stable blankets are ordinary woolen blanketing and jute sacking lined with stout woolen collar check. Probably a better blanket than this is one made of extra heavy white canvas or ducking; a blanket of this kind will not permit of any cold winds striking the animals, and are very

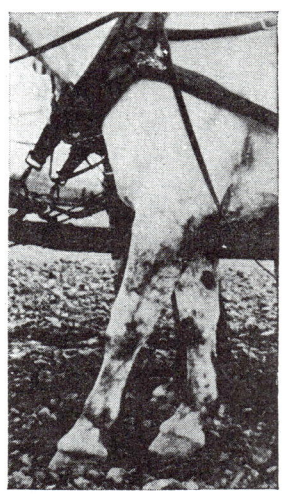

This grey horse is pointing his left front foot, which is an indication of lameness. *Courtesy Prof. R. S. Hudson, Michigan State College.*

easily kept clean owing to their hard smooth surface. A blanket or cover of this kind lined with ordinary woolen blanketing would be much warmer than the average blanket, and no doubt quite a little more expensive as well.

In fancy show horses a pad and roller are used to

fasten the blanket in place and a hood is used for the head and neck. The common type of blanket fastens directly in front on the breasts by a strap and buckle, or snap and ring; two surcingles are sewed on to keep the blanket in place, and they are either buckled or fastened with a special fastener on the order of a snap or hook. To facilitate the keeping of the blanket on the animal a "fillet string" may be placed around the quarters; this is nothing more or less than a string extending from one side of the blanket to the other, around the quarters, much the same as the breeching, only being placed a little higher upon the quarters.

The Fit of the Blanket

The blanket should fit the neck very much the same as a collar; if it is too large in the neck, the blanket does not retain its shape and is very difficult to keep in place. It should extend well down to the elbows and backward to the dock, fitting the animal rather loosely. Both the fillet string and the surcingle should be adjustable, and in fastening the surcingle, the fastener should be placed high enough that the animal will not lie on it when lying down.

The blankets should be shaken quite often, and brushed occasionally to remove the loose hair and the dirt that collects on them. If it becomes necessary to wash them use cold water and just as little soap as possible. It sometimes becomes necessary due to contagious diseases and skin ailments to disinfect the blankets; cold disinfectant solutions should be used and the blanket stretched at intervals during the time that it is drying.

The Use and Abuse of Blankets

Blankets should not be used in the fall until the temperature requires them for the comfort of the animal and then only for warmth. It is a very common mistake made by some horsemen to keep the barn very tight and close, and then blanket their horses very heavily to induce the accumulation of excessive fat and to make them exceedingly sleek. This lowers the vitality of the animals and renders them quite liable to diseases induced by exposure to inclement weather. The ventilation of the barn should always be ample to keep the air pure and eliminate the moisture. Horses never suffer from cold in a well ventilated barn, as the moisture is always removed before it has become cold enough to make its influence felt upon the animals. The use of a blanket under the harness, or on the outside, during very cold weather should never be permitted while the animal is working. This is a common practice but one to be condemned under all conditions.

Bedding the Horse

When the animal is brought to the stable excessively sweaty or wet, it should be dried with rubbers,

STABLE CLOTHING AND BEDDING 41

until the excess of moisture has been eliminated; the animal must not be blanketed while in an extremely wet condition, but should be allowed to dry somewhat, first. It should be blanketed, however, before it gets cold enough to show a reaction to the temper-

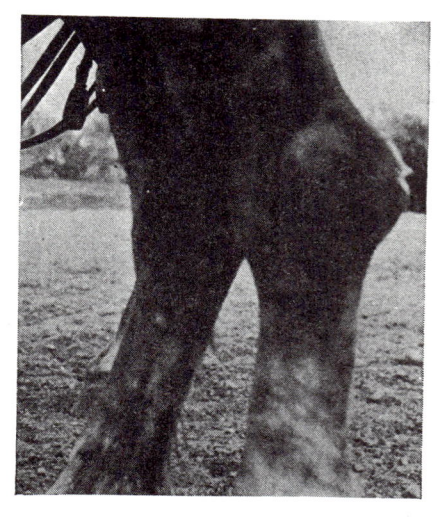

This horse has a capped hock. Often caused by kicking against the stable walls. *Courtesy Prof. R. S. Hudson, Michigan State College.*

ature by shivering. If the blanket is placed on the animal while the coat is excessively wet, it will absorb a quantity of the moisture and the dampness of the blanket will only make the animal more uncomfortable and add to the possibilities of producing a reaction that will be detrimental to the animal.

The Purposes of Bedding

By providing a good bed for the horse, we are but practicing economy in his management. While it is true that most horses take much of their rest while standing, and that there are others that rarely lie down, yet the providing of a good comfortable bed may do much toward inducing them to take some rest at least, lying down. We are very positive that with most horses, a good bed influences them to rest much of the time lying down, to save their legs, and if the bed is properly made it protects them from injuries on the hard floor.

A good bed for the horse should be level, dry and warm, should absorb or allow the urine to drain away in its entirety, and have no injurious actions upon the hoofs or the body. Most materials have some objections but we do have several that can be used very successfully when properly managed. While straw is a common material used for bedding, and by far the most common, as well as the most satisfactory, yet we have other materials that can be used when circumstances make it necessary; the most common of these are saw-dust, shavings, sand and leaves.

Straw as a Bedding Material

Straw to make the best bed should be long, dry, clean, free from mold and of a good bright color. The majority of straw that is used for bedding has been baled and this crushes it to such an extent that it does not produce as good a bed as the whole unbaled straw. Straw makes a very attractive bed when properly prepared, being clean and bright looking and very elastic. However, for the best results enough straw should always be available to keep the soiled straw replaced at all times. A thick wet urine soaked mass of straw in the bedding is very unsanitary and should not be permitted under any conditions.

It requires some little experience to make up a bed properly; in the first place the straw must be laid criss-crossed, for if it is laid straight it does not make a good bed, and does not remain in place long. Where the horses stand in a single stall the bedding should not be placed too far forward, as the horse usually lies as far back in his stall as his tie strap will permit. In making up the bed the straw should be patted down with the fork to get it neatly arranged; if it is left too fluffy and loose it will be moved into large masses by the movement of the animal's feet. We know of no better way for the average horseman to secure the few little practical details that are necessary in making a suitable bed for the horse, than to watch the caretaker or swipe prepare the bed of one of our modern race horses.

The bedding should be removed from the stall, or at least from in under the animal's feet during the day; the wet and urine soaked straw should be removed as well as all of the manure. If the bedding is but slightly soiled it can be used again after it has been dried. It should be piled in such a way that the air will circulate through it and dry it out thoroughly. There is objection to throwing the bedding to the front of the stall; a greedy horse may eat it and he will be compelled to breathe the strong ammonia fumes from any of it that may be soaked with urine. The best way to handle it, is to throw it in a pile at the rear of the stall out of the reach of the animal's feet. New straw can be added to the straw from time to time, as it may be needed.

Wheat straw is no doubt the best straw that is used for bedding; it is long, tough, hard and will wear well; it is not as sweet as oat straw and not so readily eaten. It should be of a bright yellow color.

Oat straw is more easily crushed and will not wear as long as wheat straw; it is sweeter to the taste and is easily digested, so horses are apt to eat it quite greedily.

Rye straw is the best of all the straws as it is longest and toughest; however, it is too high priced and in too great demand for stuffing collars and other purposes. The straw is smaller than wheat straw and not so bright in color.

Barley straw is not suitable for bedding the horse as the awns on the head may irritate the skin, and if eaten in any great quantity may cause colic.

Leaves would make a very good bed and one that is very economical. It is doubtful if horsemen would very often be compelled to resort to the use of such material, as they can usually procure bedding material of some kind. They could be used in case nothing better could be secured. They do not drain the urine away as well as we would like.

The Use of Sawdust

Sawdust may be used for bedding horses, but it should not be used unless ample supplies are available as it ferments very rapidly. The sawdust should be from well seasoned logs; if it is from green timber it will become heated as soon as it is packed into a bed and soaked with urine, and will cause an irritation of the skin; it is not an unusual sight to see animals that are bedded with sawdust have a large scabby surface, where they have lain with that part of the skin next to the heated sawdust. If there are drains in the stable they should be stopped up, before sawdust is used, or it will wash into them and clog them. The sawdust must be removed as soon as it is soiled or wet with urine. In very hot weather if allowed to remain damp, it may become flyblown and full of maggots.

Shavings make a very good bed, where they can be secured; they do not heat so badly as sawdust and are not as absorbent. They do contain some large blocks of wood, which should be removed by hand. The same precautions in handling it as in the use of sawdust should be taken.

Sand as a Bedding Material

Sand may be used in a dry hot climate, and where the floor is not damp; it should never be used in damp cold climates. Care must be taken that the sand is free from all traces of salt, or the horses may eat large quantities of it, which will produce a serious, if not a fatal colic.

The practice of allowing the bedding to remain under the animal all the time, is not to be recommended. It gradually works to the rear of the animal and in a short time we find that it is simply a damp heap; it is very unsanitary and should be condemned for this purpose.

Before using any absorbent bedding stop all the drains to prevent them from being clogged. As a general practice do not bed the animal down until he has been cleaned, and as the horse will usually stale as soon as the bed is placed under him it is well to place a small fork full of soiled bedding under it, and then remove it when the bedding down is performed for the night; this conserves bedding material.

CHAPTER IV

STABLE TRICKS AND VICES OF THE HORSE

Probably there are few horsemen but who have had the privilege of observing in some horses one or more of the vices or tricks that they are commonly subject to. The disadvantages of horses afflicted with any one of the many tricks and vices are loss of condition in the animal, danger in handling on account of injury and the annoyance that they cause, and in some cases the destruction of stable equipment and clothing. Most of these conditions are acquired from association with other animals, while a few may be the result of some disease or injury and others may result from unkind treatment.

If one is buying an animal from one who has owned it for some time, it is always well to first observe the horse in the stall; pass in beside it, noting its action and behavior. If it is a work animal it is well to observe the harnessing operation. Observe the manger for evidence of cribbing and the sides and back of the stall for evidence of kicking; if in the winter, make an effort to observe the clothing, to determine whether the animal tears it or not. It might be well to use the comb and brush for a few minutes to detect any difficulty. in grooming. Careful notice should be taken of the animal while being hitched. There are very few tricks and vices but what detract very much from the animal's value, and some of them are so serious as to make the ani-

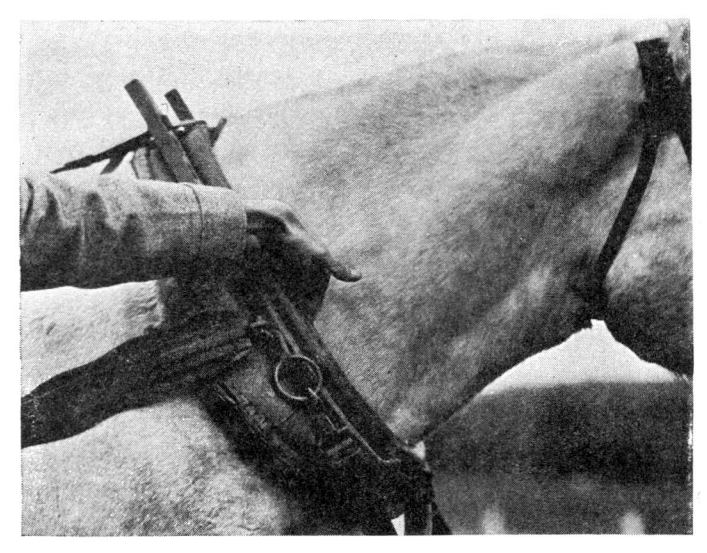

The collar should buckle at the top and one should be able to insert the flat hand between the horse's neck and the collar at the sides. *Courtesy Prof. R. S. Hudson, Michigan State College.*

mal almost useless for work purposes, while others render it dangerous to handle the animal.

If animals are kept out of doors as much as possible when not in use, it will lessen the liability of learning these tricks. It is also good for the animal as it provides much needed exercise. Idleness with the greater part of the time spent in the stable is conducive to disease, as well as the possible acquiring of tricks and vices.

The Habit of Weaving

This is a habit that is noticed very often in race horses and especially in wild animals in captivity. The animal will weave back and forth continually and at times to the extent that the feet will alternately be raised and lowered to the floor with the movements of the body. This is a nervous condition that may be brought about by some disease condition; however, there is not as far as we know any particular disease that has been credited with producing this habit. It is very possible, however, that this condition may be started in an animal from observing another animal.

Some horses weave constantly, while others weave only a part of the time; it is needless to state that any animal practicing this habit continually is greatly weakened and incapacitated for work. It requires too much energy during the constant weaving. Such animals should always be kept apart from others so that they do not contract the habit from observance. They should be provided with bedding that will not slip under them and should be placed in a large roomy box stall. If possible, they should be allowed to run in the pasture for some little time, or as much of the time as the weather will permit.

The extent to which the animal is affected by the

habit will determine the disposition of it. If it renders it weak and unable to work it should be destroyed. If it can work without much inconvenience, and will remain in fairly good flesh while doing so, it may be used in this way.

Windsucking and Crib-Biting

These are by far the most common habits that we find amongst work horses. They lower the selling value of many a good horse to a ridiculous figure, and at the best are very undesirable. However, many of these animals are capable of giving very satisfactory service for years, with no other inconvenience to the owner, than the time and bother of attending to the method of constantly preventing the performance of the act.

A windsucker arches its neck, draws its head toward the breast and gives a gulp, thus swallowing air. The crib-biter accomplishes the same end, but it catches hold of the manger or some other object in order to get a good purchase, and at the time it pulls back a grunt is emitted.

A windsucker cannot be recognized but the cribbiter can be recognized by its worn off teeth. In some animals these teeth are worn down almost to the gums. Colic or indigestion frequently result from this habit.

There is no question but what horses will learn both of these habits from observing horses, and for

STABLE TRICKS AND VICES 51

this reason horses that have acquired these habits should be kept away from all other horses. Many methods have been used to prevent this practice of horses, but many times they outwit the device. They usually desist during the time that the act produces

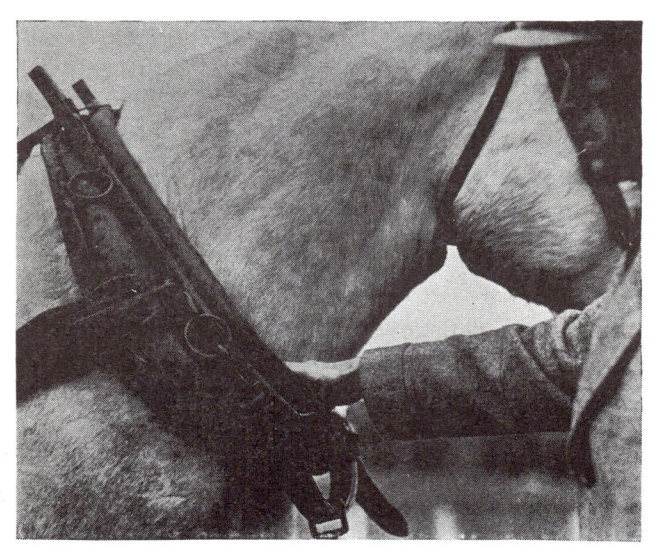

The collar should be long enough that you can insert the hand between it and the underside of the horse's neck. *Courtesy Prof. R. S. Hudson, Michigan State College.*

any discomfort, but as soon as they find a way to practice the habit without any discomfort they are performing the act as of old. Many of the practices that were used were cruel and should not be countenanced at all. Sawing between the teeth, lacing wire between the teeth at the gums, are both cruel and last only as long as the soreness lasts. One of the best methods is to take a wide strap and place around the neck just back of the region where the throat lash rests. This should be buckled tight enough so that the horse cannot arch his neck. This will not interfere with breathing, eating or drinking; it should be removed when the horse is working, unless he cribs on the yoke or tongue, and in such cases it may be worn at all times. Muzzles have been tried, but are not as satisfactory as the wide strap. The horse may be placed in a stall with four blank walls and fed from the floor, but as this will not prevent windsucking it is not as practical as the use of the strap. Horses have been known to crib on the toe of a front foot, so the blank walls would not answer all cases even for a crib-biter. Always remove from the other horses. No permanent cure has been found to date.

Kicking in the Stable

This is a very serious habit as it is apt to injure the animal, destroy the stall, and besides is very annoying. This habit is no doubt worse in mares than geldings; it is practiced most often by the animals when they are idle. Spending the greater part of their time in the open is a good method of preventing this habit.

There are many methods of trying to prevent this habit, but none of them will absolutely prevent it. Padding the portions of the stall that are being

STABLE TRICKS AND VICES

struck by the animal, hanging sacks of sand, dirt, etc., where the animal may strike them when kicking, hanging prickly bushes so that they may be struck, and the buckling of a short piece of leather around the ankle to which is fastened a short piece of chain, that will strike the legs when the animal kicks. If no other means will do the legs may be shackled together. Some animals kick only when the stable is dark; hanging a light in the barn will prevent some horses from kicking. When any of these methods are used, by which the animal can injure itself, careful attention must be given that such injury does not occur.

Crowding in the Stall

This is a very dangerous habit as far as the attendant is concerned. This consists of the animals forcing the attendant against the side of the stall and holding him there by crowding against him. It is frequently that ribs are broken in this way, or that a foot is mashed by the animals trampling upon it. This habit is found more often in mares than in geldings, and often during the heat period. Careless handling and roughness during grooming and soreness of the neck or shoulders may all be the cause of the acquiring of this habit. In some animals this habit is only noticed during grooming or harnessing, in others at any time.

If the animal is very bad it may be necessary to place it in a wide stall and then to place a pole in the

54 SOME COMMON DISEASES OF THE HORSE

stall, and fasten at the manger far enough from the wall so that the attendant can walk in behind it.

Biting

Occasionally mares and geldings in a playful way will bite the attendant during grooming; this is quite painful as though they did it with malicious intent, so it should never be encouraged by tickling with the brush or comb, or any unnecessary procedure. It may be the result of careless grooming of tender skinned animals, or improper handling of an animal with a sore neck or sore shoulders. If the animal is very vicious a muzzle may be used at all times except during the feeding period. In others the use of a side stick will do very well; it is simply a stick one end of which is fastened in the nose band of the halter and the other to a surcingle around the body.

Tearing the Clothing

This is one habit that some horses acquire that is very apt to try the owner's patience. It is one that as a rule is very hard to control with any satisfaction. It is doubtful if it can be prevented successfully when once fully acquired. The best method of prevention is by the use of a stout leather guard which is fastened to the halter strap that passes under the horse's jaw. This strap must be long enough to reach below the lips and then the animal cannot get hold of the clothing; a muzzle can also be used, but must be kept in place during the time the blanket is worn.

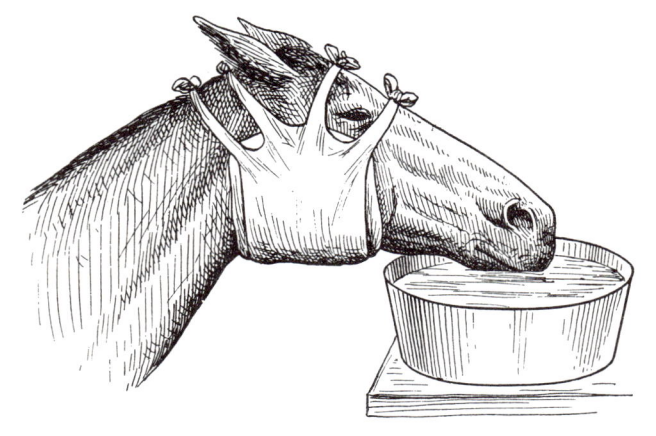

This is a satisfactory method of applying a poultice to a horse with a sore throat.

Gnawing the Walls

This is an indication usually that the animal requires some minerals, such as lime; many times a lump of rock salt in the feed box or a regular supply of salt will remedy the trouble. When this does not secure the desired results the walls may be painted with creosote or tar, with some creolin or other objectionable substance added.

Eating Manure

This is a very dirty habit, and when once acquired is often very difficult to get stopped; it many times is an indication of improper feed, or it may be that of indigestion. With this habit it is always advisable to have a thorough veterinary examination of the animal made as soon as possible.

CHAPTER V

GROOMING THE HORSE

Relation of Grooming to Exercise

The statement that a horse that is working is much easier to clean than an idle one may seem out of place, nevertheless it is true, as careful observation and study will prove. An idle horse is always hard to keep clean, and some horses' skin is extremely difficult to be kept free from scurf and grease. This accumulation is always greater when an animal is stall fed than when he is running at grass. It no doubt is one of those wise provisions of Nature that provides for the removing of the dirt and the accumulations of excretions from the skin by the workings of the natural elements and the feeding of Nature's best animal food, grass. We conclude from this that exercise, or work, is not only beneficial to the health of the animal by keeping the organs functioning properly, but it also saves labor for the groom.

All horses that are used for work of any kind are kept under purely unnatural conditions. For this reason animals from whom it is expected that the maximum amount of work is to be secured must have a goodly amount of grooming, which should consist of brushing and rubbing. In the natural state the horse eats just enough food to maintain his bodily needs and takes just enough exercise to carry him from one grazing spot to another. In the stable, as fed by man, he receives much more feed than his

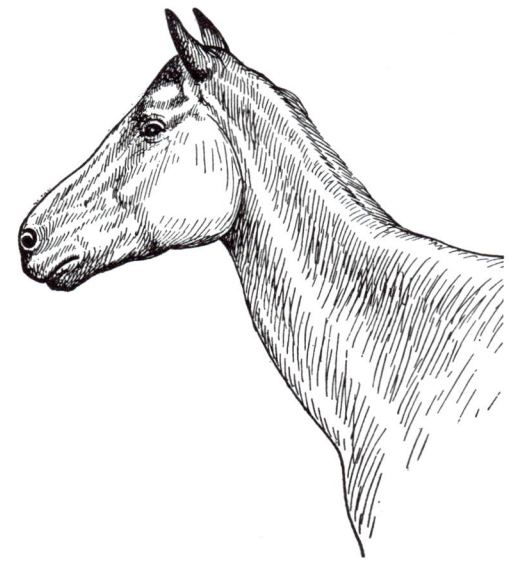

This shows a horse with a ewe neck—a somewhat common faulty conformation in horses.

body requires for its own building up and maintenance, and this extra amount is converted into energy for the production of the work that man has intended that he should do. The digestive organs are called upon to handle this extra amount of feed, and in the course of the work that is performed the various organs of the body provide for the elimination of the greatly increased amount of waste products that are sure to result from the digestion of this extra amount of food. The lungs, intestines, kidneys and skin must eliminate this waste. It is an obvious fact, then, that when it is desired that the horse must perform difficult, fast work that one of the best methods of keeping the body fit is by thorough grooming.

Grooming Tools

While we are aware of the fact that the average horseman cannot, as a common practice, spend a lot of time to groom dirt from the hair, for this purpose the bristle brushes are better than fiber brushes; for, while the fiber brush does very well at first, it soon flattens down and the fibers will not penetrate the hair. The bristles will wear off, but will not flatten down. It is well to keep in mind that as the bristles get shorter in a bristle brush that they become stiffer, and in using on a thin-skinned horse care must be used.

Curry Combs and Their Use

The common type of curry comb is made from several blunt-toothed blades; others are circular and are very flexible, being made from light spring steel; they also have blunt teeth. One of the best types, however, is the humane curry comb, which consists of a number of circular cup-shaped pieces of metal arranged in consecutive circles and having no teeth;

60 SOME COMMON DISEASES OF THE HORSE

the edges of these cups, which are on a level with each other, is simply crumpled, or creased. This cleans the hair very well and there are no teeth to injure the animal's skin. The reason for having the teeth of the curry comb blunt is to prevent wearing

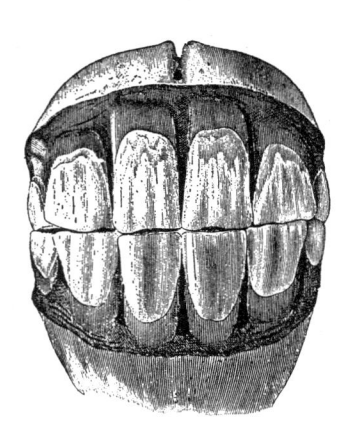

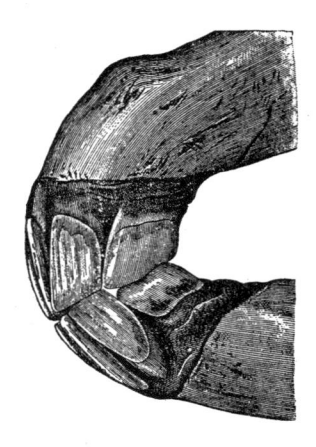

This shows the incisor teeth of a young horse—the teeth are wide and flat and meet at almost right angle.

away the bristles of the brush and injuring the skin of the horse. The back of the curry comb is fitted with a loop of webbing, or strap, to enable its being held in the hand. Some of them are fitted with small projections for the purpose of dislodging the dirt that collects in them by striking them against the stall, or the floor. Some patterns have a straight wooden handle.

The use of the curry comb is very much abused and is the best liked grooming tool for lazy men, as

GROOMING THE HORSE

it makes possible a quick grooming. It should not be used much upon the animal's body, never upon the head, or upon the legs, except that it may be used to remove dirt that cannot be brushed off the legs. Its greatest use should be for cleaning the body brush. It does enable the much quicker grooming, where it is employed for the entire body, and in some thick, heavy coated, thick-skinned horses it may do no particular harm to use it. In cleaning the dirt from the comb it should be dislodged by knocking it on the floor behind the horse. It is a dirty practice and unsanitary to blow the dirt from the comb, or to strike against the stall at some little distance from the floor, thus allowing the dirt to become circulated in the air of the stable to be breathed by both man and beast.

The Water Brush

It is made of longer, finer and more flexible bristles than the body brush; it is used mostly for wetting the mane and tail, also for washing the feet. It is, however, a fine brush for cleaning the head and face. It may also serve for a thin-skinned, ticklish horse that has a light coat.

The Dandy Brush

It is made of coarse, heavy thick fiber. It should only be used for removing the mud from the legs, but as the bristles are stiff it penetrates the hair very readily, and in stables where a quick grooming is desired it is usually used in conjunction with the curry comb. Their chief advantage is that they save both time and labor.

Sponges

Are used about the head in cleaning the eyes, face and nostrils. The greatest objection to sponges is the fact that infection is very apt to be carried from one animal to another by their use. At the first sign of any disease among the horses, they should be discarded. They cannot be disinfected by boiling as this ruins them. Their greatest objection then is the fact that they are very unsanitary.

Rubbers or Rubbing Cloths

A rubber simply consists of a fair sized piece of cloth that is used to give the horse's coat a good polish. Should be of the most convenient size to be easily handled. The best ones no doubt are those made from salt sacks. Can be wet and used for the same purpose as the sponge. Can be disinfected by boiling. The use of the rubber greatly improves the appearance of the coat.

The Sweat Scraper

There are two kinds in common use. The one that has a flexible blade and the other is a stiff blade made of wood or aluminum and is slightly curved; it

GROOMING THE HORSE 63

is claimed that the flexible one gives the best satisfaction as it conforms to the curves of the body and the limbs. The sweat scraper is used to remove the sweat and lather from the horse; it may also be used for removing the water and mud from the horse's legs. It saves time and labor in removing the excess of water from the coat of the horse. They are not really necessary in work horse stables but in certain cases they may be of value, especially if horses are being prepared for showing.

Mane Combs and Their Uses

They are made of horn or metal with rather deep coarse teeth. They can be gotten along without in the average stable but they are of considerable value when properly used. They are for cleaning and straightening the hairs in the mane and tail.

Time for Grooming

The best time for grooming is at the close of the day's work unless the work has been very exhaustive and the animal is very tired; in this case it should be allowed to rest first. By giving the animal a thorough grooming at night it will need but a light grooming in the morning, simply to remove the dirt and produce a cleanly appearance.

Method of Grooming

The horse should be cool and dry. Begin grooming on the left side of the neck, immediately behind the left ear, thoroughly brushing out the coat, mov-

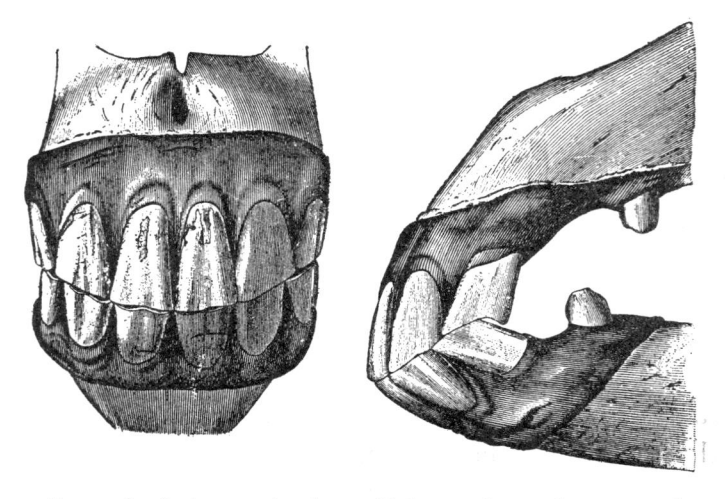

Shows the incisor teeth of an old horse—the teeth are round and the teeth come together at an oblique angle.

ing the brush in the direction that the hair lies; if dirt is excessive and sticks rather close, it may be necessary to move the brush in a circular direction. To use the brush to the best advantage it is advisable to stand at some distance from the horse, about arm's length, and holding the arm fairly rigid, lean a portion of the body right against the brush, thus forcing it through the hair. The brush should not be brought down with too much force upon the skin of those animals which have a tender skin. If the operator stands too close to the animal and with his arm bent, he is not as apt to remove the dirt so effectively as the bristles do not penetrate the coat. After the one side is completed, the other side is groomed in the same manner, starting at the same place on the neck. The legs can be groomed at the time the sides are groomed, or they may be finished after the body is completed. At this stage of the grooming, if you desire to do a good job, turn the animal around in the stall to clean the face, eyes and nostrils. It is much more convenient and you can do a much better job of it as the manger is in your way if you do this part of the grooming with the animal standing in the stall naturally. The animal is again turned in the stall and the mane and tail are brushed out, and the animal is given the final polish with the rubber.

Use a soft brush or a rubber for cleaning the head; a dry water brush is as good as anything you can use. Do not knock the skin or the bony projections on the head and legs while grooming them.

Brushing the Mane

The hair should be brushed until well separated, and then taking a lock at a time, beginning at the highest point of the withers, brush out each lock separately. The purpose of starting at the withers is

66 SOME COMMON DISEASES OF THE HORSE

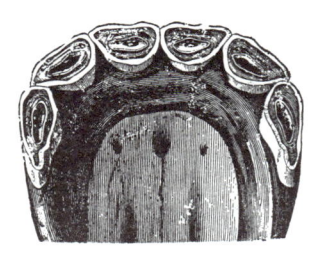

Upper Front Teeth at Nine
Years of Age

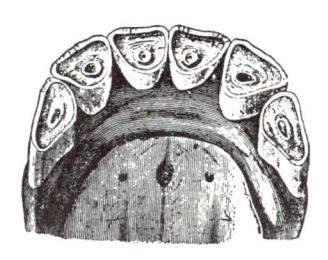

Upper Front Teeth at Fifteen
Years of Age

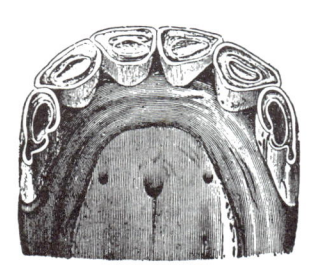

Upper Front Teeth at Ten
Years of Age

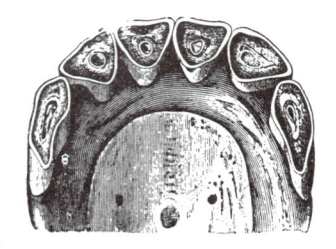

Upper Front Teeth at Twenty-
One Years of Age

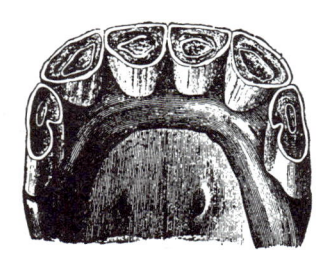

Upper Front Teeth at Eleven
Years of Age

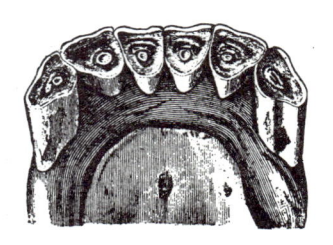

Upper Front Teeth at Thirty
Years of Age

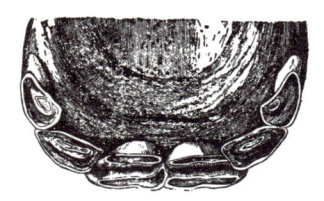

Lower Front Teeth at Three
Years of Age

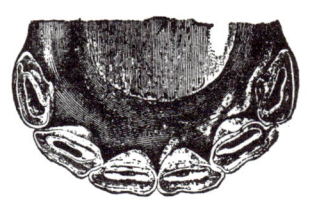

Lower Front Teeth at Six
Years of Age

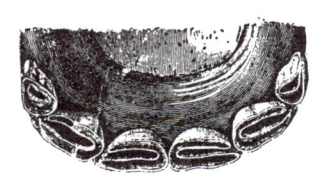

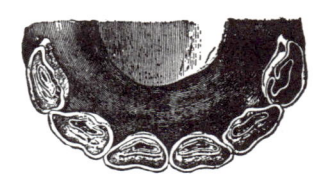

Lower Front Teeth at Four
Years of Age

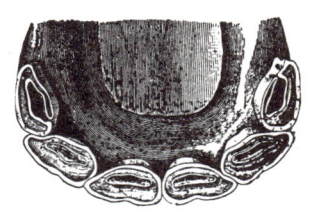

Lower Front Teeth at Seven
Years of Age

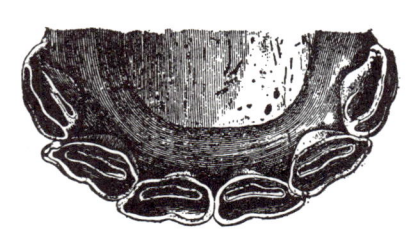

Lower Front Teeth at Five
Years of Age

Lower Front Teeth at Eight
Years of Age

the prevention of the dirtying of that part that has previously been cleaned.

Thinning Mane

This can only be done properly when the hair has been thoroughly brushed and should only be done when the mane is too heavy and thick to be kept in good condition. This is accomplished best by taking a few hairs at a time from the under surface and freeing them from the rest of the hair and removing them with a quick jerk. The hair on the outside of the mane should not be touched at all. When the mane has been sufficiently thinned it should be brushed out thoroughly, and any portions that are too long can be removed by plucking them out with the fingers. They should not be clipped as this spoils the appearance of the mane.

Laying the Mane

This can usually be accomplished by brushing the mane thoroughly with a wet brush. If this does not accomplish the desired effect, the mane may be wetted and then braided in small locks. If neither of these methods are satisfactory the mane may be plastered down by wet clay, which will wash out very well when dry. It may take several applications of clay.

CHAPTER VI

HOW TO HANDLE THE HORSE

Most horses are very tractable and easily handled, yet there are times when due to some diseased or injured condition affecting them, it becomes necessary to restrain them. In restraining the horse, it is done for the purpose of insuring safety to the attendant and to enable the attendant to perform the necessary duty, whatever it may be; in some cases animals must be restrained to prevent them injuring themselves.

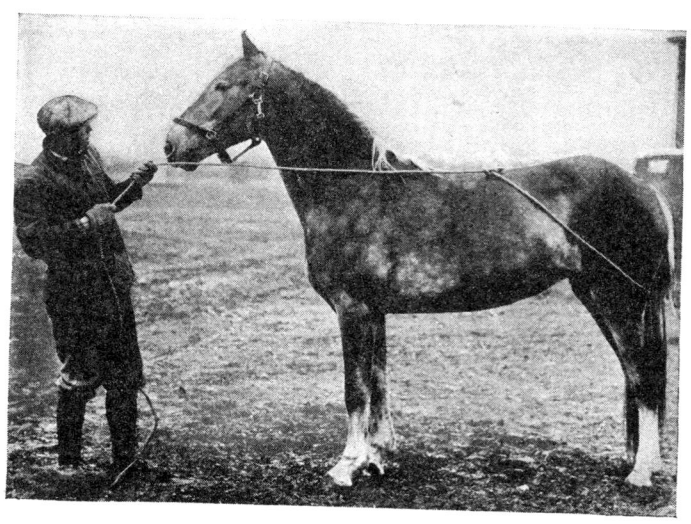

A very good method to use when breaking a colt to lead. Also useful when first tying the colt in the stable.

There are many special methods and appliances for restraining the horse, but for our purposes, we are interested only in those methods that can be utilized in any stable. No method of restraint should be used that is liable to injure the animal. Methods of restraint that produce considerable pain should be employed as little as possible.

There are three methods of restraint in common use; the use of an implement producing pain, thus occupying the animal's attention during the period that the pain is caused. The use of mechanical means to render the animal immobile and the use of anæsthetics which render the animal unconscious. The first two only concern us, and various methods are in use. In far too many instances, methods of restraint are used, that are really not necessary. It should be the policy of the good horseman to use such means just as little as possible. There is a very noticeable difference in men's ability to handle animals during a variety of circumstances and under a wide range of conditions. The horse is a creature of memory and quite often a firm hold of the reins and a stern command from the attendant is all that is needed in a great many instances.

The Use of the Twitch

The most common and the most widely used method of restraining the horse. It is very successful and the ease and rapidity with which it can be used accounts for its being universally used by horsemen the world over. It is used too many times when it really isn't needed due to the reasons just mentioned. It consists of a small rope or a piece of latigo leather, tied so as to form a small loop, just large enough to fit over the horse's upper lip; to this there is a handle

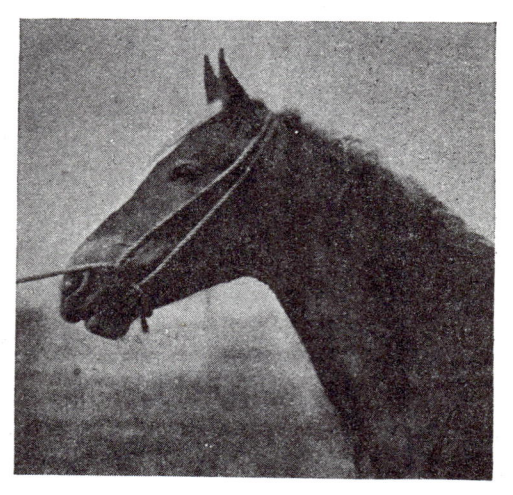

A good type of war bridle for use in controlling a horse that requires it.

fitted for twisting this loop after it has been put into the proper position. This handle can be of any material just so it accomplishes the desired results; usually it is a short piece of wood, say from 12 to 24 inches long, that has a small hole in one end just large enough for the rope to pass through; the rope is placed through this hole and the ends fastened to form the loop.

The loop should be placed around the wrist of the left hand. The operator grasps the halter of the horse with the right hand if he is working alone, but if he has an assistant he permits him to hold the animal; in such a case his right hand is placed across the animal's nose to steady the head; with the left hand grasp the upper lip; release the hold of the right hand and slip the loop over the left hand and over the lip; with the right hand grasp the handle of the twitch, tightening it up by twisting it. It is best to make twitches small, for if they are made too large, the operator is quite likely to injure the animal by using too much force. The twitch can also be used upon the animal's ear in cases where for any reason it is not desired to use it on the nose. In no case should the twitch be used unless it is necessary and then never apply enough force to injure the animal. If the twitch is to be used for any length of time, it should be removed often or it may produce an injury to the parts. It will also prevent the animal from getting restless.

The War and Pulley Bridle

These, like the twitch, are instruments of torture, and are much used in the control of mean or vicious horses. They should never be used unless it is absolutely necessary. There are several ways that these two bridles can be made, but the principles are the same, and for that reason we will give you these

HOW TO HANDLE THE HORSE

methods that are easiest and most cheaply constructed. For making either of these, a piece of ⅜ inch rope about 25 to 30 feet long and a small pulley is needed. This rope should be strong and of good quality. To make a pulley bridle, take the rope and fasten the pulley on one end and then pass the loose

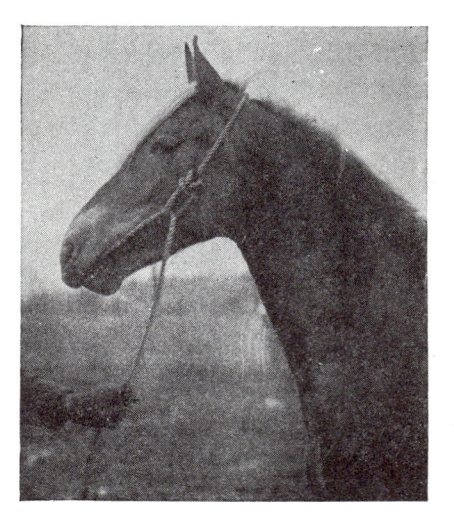

Another type of war bridle. Very satisfactory when needed.

end through the pulley until a loop about the diameter equal to the length of the horse's head remains; put the loop in the animal's mouth as you should a bridle bit and then over the top of the head; the pulley should rest on one side of the head below the ear or any other location down to slightly below the eye; the pulley should be on the piece of rope passing over the top of the head, for then when traction is applied the loop will tighten and remain in position. This is a very effectual method of holding a mean or vicious horse. It can be used very success-

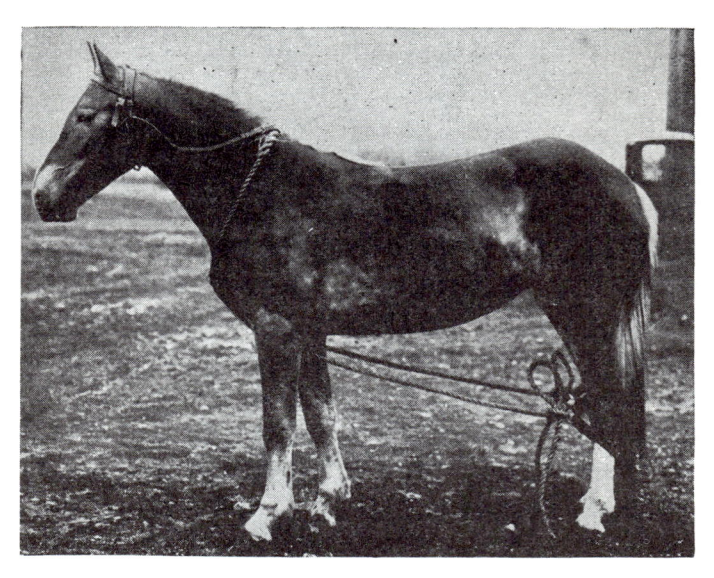

A satisfactory hopple to control kicking horse. Also used as a breeding hopple.

fully for a horse that has the habit of breaking loose while being led.

The war bridle works on about the same principle; the simplest way is to loop the rope about the animal's neck and fasten by tying just as snug as possible without interfering with the movements of the neck; then take the loose end of the rope and pass it through this loop around the neck until the loop resulting is about 12 to 15 inches in diameter; place this loop in the animal's mouth the same as a bit and draw taut. Used the same as the pulley bridle. Most horses can be controlled by either of these. Neither of them should be used unless it is absolutely necessary.

Taking Up the Fore-Leg

This may be done in one of two ways; by taking a broad strong strap and holding up either of the front feet while it is looped once around the fore-arm; the long end is then passed around the cannon in the region of the fetlock and passed through the buckle and drawn quite snug. Another method is by taking a long rope and passing over the horse's back and around the body (this making about $1\frac{1}{2}$ turns about the body) and by fastening the loose end of the rope to the foot in the region of the pastern and then pulling it up against the body by traction on the end of the tops on the opposite side of the body; rope should be 25 to 30 feet long and about $\frac{3}{8}$ or $\frac{1}{2}$ inch in diameter.

Either of these methods are of value where an animal strikes or kicks. They do not injure the animal and are easily and quickly used.

Squeeze or Crowding

Horses with sore necks and shoulders are often very difficult to handle, and due to the liability to injury, it is necessary that they be controlled in some way. If it is desired to treat them in the stable, we know of no better way than to secure a long pole and crowd the animal to one side of the stall, fasten the end to the hay rack or to any strong fixture, pressing it

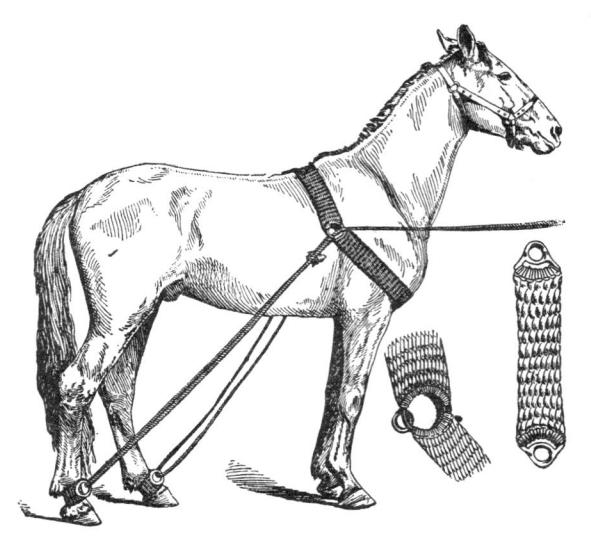

A casting harness for throwing a horse for castration and other purposes.

against the animal quite snugly. The other end can be moved toward the horse and it can be crowded up very closely against the side of the stall. This reduces the danger from injury to the minimum and does no harm the horse. The front of the pole should be fastened at a height of the shoulders and the rear end upon a level with the stifle joint; should not be too low; when using this the horse should be securely tied with a strong halter.

If the pole is not suitable and the barnyard should happen to have a very strong gate that opens back against the fence, it is often possible to stand the horse in the triangular space made when the gate is opened back and crowd it against the fence; this method cannot safely be used unless the fence is made of lumber and it must be strong.

Both of these methods are very good for the dressing of sore necks, shoulders or backs or in the treating of fistula of the withers.

The Side Line

This is a rope that is used to take up one of the hind legs; it is used by tying a large loop in one end of a rope and placing it about the animal's neck and then placing the loose end around the pastern of the hind foot that is to be taken up and then pass upward through the loop at the neck; traction is then applied upon the loose end of the rope and the foot is drawn upward and forward; to eliminate pressure upon the windpipe the long end should be passed between the forelegs before it is placed about the hind foot. This is a very useful way to handle horses that kick while being harnessed. Care should be taken that the heels are not chafed by the rope. The larger the rope, the less liable this is to happen.

There are many other methods of restraint, but when it is not possible to control the animal with the methods outlined here, it is advisable to secure a competent and experienced man that has the necessary apparatus for handling such animals.

CHAPTER VII

CLIPPING THE HORSE

The Winter Coat

Under natural conditions the coat of the horse becomes heavy and thick for the winter season; it is Nature's way of protecting the animal from the cold and assisting the animal in maintaining its normal body weight. This was the season of the year that horses under natural conditions were very short of food, hence the advisability of maintaining their body weight. The warmth is not all from the long furry coat, but during the cold months idle horses are not, as a general rule, groomed very often, and there is a very pronounced greasiness occurring in the coat, which also aids in keeping the animal warm.

It is a well known fact that the hair of draft horses is naturally coarse, as compared to that of the finely bred horses. However, the better bred the animal is the finer the coat, with the exception of the mane and tail hair, which is always permanent; the horse's coat is changed twice each year. It changes to thick coat in the fall for the winter season and to a fine one in the summer. Horses are not considered in their best physical condition at this time, and this is a very critical time in their care if it is desired to keep them

80 SOME COMMON DISEASES OF THE HORSE

in the best condition. The hair that is shed is sometimes spoken of as temporary hair. The average draft horse will yield from 7 to 8 pounds of hair, dirt and dandruff by clipping; harness horses do not have

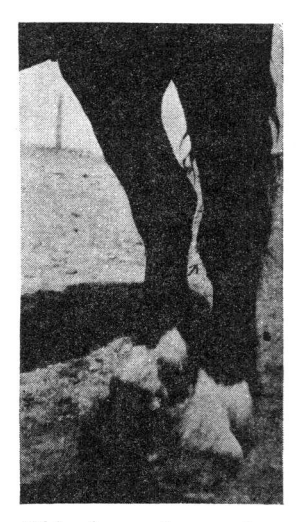

This horse has a bog spavin. Do not use such horses for breeding. *Courtesy Prof. R. S. Hudson, Michigan State College.*

as heavy coat of hair as draft horses; the mane and tail contain about 1-½ pounds. It is of no value, but it may be interesting to know that the ordinary hair of horse is about 4,300 to the square inch.

Nature has provided very wisely for the comfort of the horse, so that with the approach of cold weather the coat responds by becoming longer, and with the

CLIPPING THE HORSE

approach of spring the animal begins to shed. This will often happen upon moving an animal to a climate with a different temperature. The hair is so regulated that it will only make so much growth, and it then remains stationary. Nature has regulated this according to the season.

The horse does not always shed his coat early enough in the spring to enable him to work without sweating very freely. Horses with a heavy coat will soon get out of condition, and, to prevent this, clipping is usually resorted to.

Purpose of Clipping

If an animal must work a thick, heavy coat adds to the labor, as it produces constant sweating in the animal and does not give the hair a chance to dry out. A horse cannot work long under such conditions and maintain his body weight; it is sure to lose flesh. By clipping the horse we enable him to do more work, prevent the necessary distress of working with a covering of thick, heavy hair, the coat dries better, he is much easier cleaned and can be kept in condition. It is often practiced in horses working at a walk to clip only trace high; that is, the legs and belly only. There is a wide variety of opinion upon this subject, but we are partial to the opinion that if any clipping is to be done on the body at all that the entire body should be clipped. Experiments of clipping one-half of the animal's body and leaving the other side natural shows a difference in temperature, under the skin or sub-cutaneously of from 8 to 15 degrees F., the unclipped side being that many degrees below that of the side not clipped. From the unequal distribution of the blood in the body, due to this clipping of a part of the body, we conclude that if any part of the body is clipped that it should all be clipped.

It is also the belief of some that the hair covering the tendons on the back of the leg and the hair at the fetlock should be left to provide a natural drain for the water. Our experience has been that the more hair on the legs the more likely the legs are to become affected with grease heel or to become chafed, and surely they are much more easily kept clean when clipped.

The process of clipping enables the attendant to properly dry and clean the horse after the day's work. This can rarely be done with a horse that has a long, heavy coat of hair and that has sweated profusely during the day. Frequently they will not dry sufficiently between night and morning to make this possible. The labor-saving feature should not be lost sight of.

The Clipping Operation

The author can very well remember when power clippers were not so common and when the small hand clippers were used. This was a tedious process requiring about one day for each team. In earlier times horses were clipped with the shears and comb.

CLIPPING THE HORSE 83

Neither of these methods are used at the present time as the hand-power clippers are inexpensive and the ease with which clipping may be done and the time saved, make them so much superior to hand

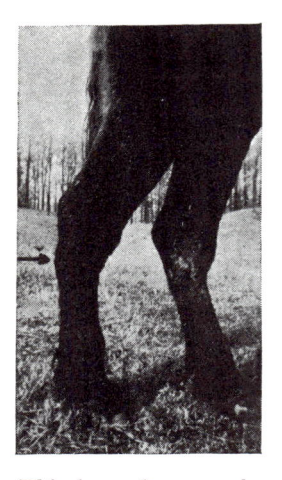

This horse has a curb. Courtesy Prof. R. S. Hudson, Michigan State College.

clippers, that we shall not consider them at all.

The blades of the clipper are made of very hard tempered material and are carefully adjusted. If great care is not used they become broken. They also clog up very easily with dirt, but not if they are dipped in kerosene oil occasionally.

The clippers should be so placed that they are not broken or overturned by any sudden movement of the animal. If the fetlock and tendon only are to be clipped they should be gradually edged off so that no ridges will show where the clipping has been done. If the legs are left unclipped the appearance is improved by slanting the cut edge from the back of the elbow upward to the front of the forearm where there is a natural dip in the limb. If the clipping is well done there will be no ridges to indicate where the clipping has been done.

The Time for the Clipping

Horses may be clipped at any time after the coat has thickened in the fall, until it shows signs of coming out in the spring. If the animals are doing hard work and kept at it steadily they may be clipped as often as the coat shows that it needs it. If the coat does not become too heavy and there is not so much to do, it will be best to clip, say about twice during the winter, about November and around New Years. It is thought by some that when an animal is clipped after the first of the year that it ruins their coat, but such is not the case. Many horses can be clipped throughout the entire year and still carry a very good appearing coat of hair. With farm horses however, one or two clippings a year will usually suffice; if there is a lot of hard work during the fall, they may be clipped in the fall and then again in the spring just before the spring work is begun. No doubt most farmers clip but once and that is in the spring.

The Effect of Winter Clipping

The horse has an unusual power of regulating his body temperature, which accounts for the fact that horses may be clipped during very cold weather, and when well fed, can even go without a blanket with impunity. However, it is not advisable to clip the horse in very cold weather without blanketing it, as it has all the appearance of cruelty and for all practical purposes, the horse that has been clipped should be protected with a blanket until the weather is warm enough that the horse will not be uncomfortable.

CHAPTER VIII

SOME CAUSES OF DISEASE IN THE HORSE

The greater percentage of ailments of the horse are those of the digestive tract. Colic or indigestion in the horse is more numerous than in any of the other of the domestic animals. When due thought and study is given to the peculiar physiological functions in the digestive system of the horse, and its peculiar anatomical construction, the causes of such conditions are easily understood.

There is no other animal that has such a small stomach in proportion to its size as does the horse. It is evident that since the stomach of the adult horse will hold but two to four gallon, that it cannot possibly hold all the feed that is consumed by the animal at one meal. It has been proved that at certain stages of digestion the food leaves the stomach of the horse as fast as it enters it. This usually prevents an impaction of the stomach. For this reason, a horse that eats too fast will either get an impaction of the stomach or will have large quantities of food thrown into the intestines before it has been sufficiently digested in the stomach. This overworks the intestines with the resulting digestive disturbances that we have so frequently in the horse.

SOME CAUSES OF DISEASE

The structure of the stomach is such that the horse cannot vomit. When food is ingested or taken into the stomach, it must pass the entire length of the intestinal tract before it gains exit from the body. In case of irritant feeds this is a very serious situation. The reason that the horse cannot vomit is due to the fact that the opening into the stomach from the gullet is very small and constricted and the lack of contact of the stomach with the abdominal walls due to its small size.

The large amount of material that is contained in the intestines is another very important factor; the horse will void excreta from seven to eight times daily, totaling in weight from thirty-five to forty pounds. In the handling of this amount of excreta, the bowels of the horse are doing a prodigious amount of work. This is one reason that pain so quickly follows even a very slight stoppage in the bowels of the horse; another is the fact that the intestines of the horse are very thin walled and easily irritated; there is none of the domestic animals in which the intestines are so easily irritated as those of the horse.

Inherited Predisposition

While we hesitate to state definitely that it is possible for the horse to inherit the susceptibility to a digestive disease, in the light of our experience we are almost compelled to do so. In treating a case of indigestion, it is not an uncommon thing to have the owner tell us that the dam of this particular animal had suffered with the same condition. We have also, when treating other kinds of diseases, heard the owner remark that the animal's dam had been attacked with the same disease at some time during her life. There cannot be much doubt but that horses inherit a weak constitution which will render them very susceptible to such diseases. We have personally had horses under our care that seem to be very susceptible to every disease that made its appearance in the neighborhood.

The weather, no doubt, plays some little part too, as disease is usually noticed to be greatly increased when a cold wet spell follows a warm dry period.

Animals of a sluggish temperament are much more susceptible to digestive diseases than high strung nervous animals.

The delicate lining of the intestines, which is so forcibly brought to our attention by the great irritation from foods or poisons and the extreme pain and rapidity with which the animal succumbs to irritation of the intestinal tract, is another important predisposing cause to disease.

General Exciting Causes

As long as the horse is permitted to roam at will and gather his feed when and where he will, and in just those amounts that his appetite calls for, we have very little trouble from disease. As soon as he is

SOME CAUSES OF DISEASE

placed under the domestication, the irregularity in habits and feeding soon manifest themselves in disease of some kind. It seems that man cannot work out the proper combination of feeding, working and rest for the horse.

The quality, quantity and manner of feeding has much to do with keeping the horse healthy; it is a well known fact that few owners feed their horses with any regard to digestive nutrients; or in many cases with very little regard to the foreign substance it contains so long as this substance is of plant origin. Feed too high in nutriment for the amount of work being done, or that contains foreign substances such as gravel and sand, etc. Feed that is moldy or spoiled. Hay that is woody and indigestible. Feeding too much and at too long intervals between feeding. Feeding in too great quantities at each feeding period, also when the animal is greatly fatigued or exhausted. No reduction of the ration during short periods of idleness, and not enough feeding periods when large quantity of feed is fed and much heavy work is being done.

The manner of watering has a decided influence upon the health of the animal; water given to horses when they are extremely hot and exhausted, may be the cause of a chill which may result in a general constitutional disturbance of a serious nature. If water is given to the horse under these conditions and the animal is not kept moving until it has cooled off, it frequently results in founder or laminitis;

given soon after the animal has eaten its meal, it is quite likely to produce some digestive disturbance, from washing the food into the intestinal tract before it has been acted upon by the digestive fluids in the stomach. When ever the horse is accustomed to any particular time, as to being watered, this custom should not be quickly changed.

Animals should never be overworked, neither should they be worked too long without food and water; they should not be compelled to perform work that is beyond their strength. Horses should not be worked too long hours, and they should be made as comfortable as possible when they are at rest.

Specific Causes of Disease

We have diseases of the horse that may affect the horse in one organ or another; we call these localized diseases and those diseases that affect the whole of the body usually through the medium of the blood stream, we call general systemic diseases. This class of diseases that I refer to are caused by germs or bacteria. Both the predisposing and the exciting causes that we have given here will assist these diseases in getting a foothold in the animal's body, due to the lowering of the vitality. Some of these diseases are contagious but all of them are infectious. Infectious diseases are those that are caused by a known infection or disease germ, but may or may not be transmitted directly from one animal to another; if it is

SOME CAUSES OF DISEASE

transmitted from one animal to another it is contagious and infectious, but if not, it is simply infectious. Tetanus or lock jaw is an infectious disease, but not contagious as it cannot be carried from one animal directly to another. Strangles, however, is a contagious infectious disease because it can be carried from one animal to another.

We have two classes of diseases that are infectious; those in which the germs produce pus and those that simply produce a poison or a toxin. Those that form pus are usually localized diseases such as strangles, etc. Those that do not are the general systemic diseases that are usually classed as blood poisons, etc. In the last named, the infection is carried to all parts of the body by the blood stream.

The germs causing disease in the horse usually gain access to the horse's body through the water that they drink, the feed they eat and the air they breathe; by far the greater part of them gain access by way of the feed and drink. Such diseases can be prevented by sanitation, that is, by the feeding of clean feeds and pure water; they can also be prevented by serums, bacterins and anti-toxins that are now being prepared for those conditions.

CHAPTER IX

HOW TO TELL THE SICK HORSE

You can only learn to tell when a horse is really sick after you have learned just how he usually acts and how he conducts himself every day. It is not out of place here to say that the horse as a usual thing cannot or at least will not, stand much pain without making considerable fuss about it. Of all the domestic animals, the horse will act strangely and queer much sooner and over a very trivial accident, injury or pain, that would not affect other farm animals.

Those persons that have had a rather wide experience with horses know quite well that the gentlest kindest horse that one can find will often become a veritable demon when suffering from an injury or from an accident, even kicking, striking and biting his attendant to whom he is usually very kind. This is very noticeable, particularly in some horses that get sore shoulders and sore necks. Other horses seem to lose all control of themselves just as soon as they receive even a slight injury. The writer has seen many horses that were almost outlaws when affected with a small sore or a slight injury. Many such horses are very kind and gentle at other times. It is always well to keep this fact in mind and use undue caution when attempting to dress an injury or sore of even the most trustworthy horse you have, for they cannot be trusted in such instances. By taking such precautions, a serious accident is often avoided.

One of the first things that is usually noticed by the attendant when the horse is ailing, is that the horse either refuses to eat or does so only sparingly. This is particularly true in digestion disturbances. The horse is usually a greedy eater and likewise loses its appetite very easily. The sick horse, unless it is with a feverish condition, usually drinks sparingly. With some conditions, especially with high fevers, the animal may drink more than usual. Most horses will drink heavily once daily in winter time unless at hard work and, occasionally, lightly in the morning. For this reason, idle farm horses, or others for that matter, can well be turned out in a paddock two or three hours after the morning meal and allowed to exercise and to drink. Water may be offered again before feeding in the evening but in very cold weather little will usually be taken.

The average horse when healthy will stool six to eight times in 24 hours or every three or four hours, when idle or at light work. Horses that are doing heavier work and that are worked faster than a walk, will frequently stool three or four times in the first two or three hours after beginning work at a moderately fast gait. Horses that are developing an impaction will frequently stool from six to eight times in two or three hours, especially when at work, but only in very small amounts. Under normal conditions, the horse will pass from 35 to 40 pounds of manure in 24 hours.

The horse that is developing an impaction or a digestive disturbance in the big bowel will frequently look around at the flank and will occasion-

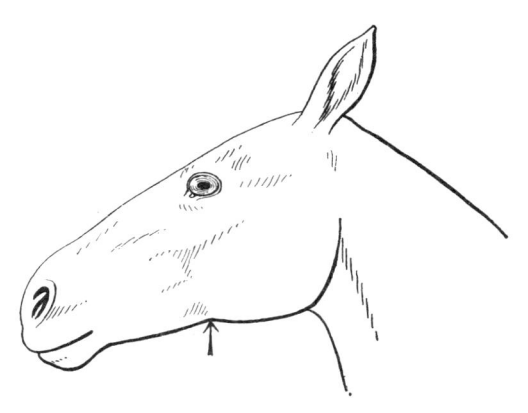

The arrow shows the location of the artery that passes over the angle of the jaw bone. By pressing the fingers against the artery you can count the horse's pulse (heart beat).

ally kick at the abdomen with the hind feet. Others will refuse to eat and show no pain at all, while still other cases will show slight colicky pains and will be restless, getting up and lying down frequently.

The rate of breathing of the horse while at rest is fairly constant, being from eight to ten times per minute and regular and rhythmical. In respiratory diseases, the rate is greatly quickened and when the rate is greatly altered as well as the manner of the animal's breathing, when the animal is at rest, it is well to begin looking for the trouble. There are many conditions that will change the animal's rate of breathing.

The pulse rate or heart beat of the well horse will vary from 36 to 40 beats per minute and this cannot be well determined unless one learns to count the beats as they can be felt in the maxillary artery, where it passes over the edge of the jaw bone just a short distance from the angle of the jaw. It only requires a little practice to learn the proper manner of making this count. The rate will not vary much in a well horse.

The temperature of the horse will vary from $98\frac{1}{2}$ to 100 degrees F., about 99 degrees F. being the average. This is usually taken by way of the rectum. The temperature of the well horse will not vary much over 1 degree F.

There are other indications that are shown by the horse during illness, but most of them are visible to the naked eye and consist only in the animal's action and behavior as it varies from the normal. The individual horse should always be studied carefully for external causes, such as poorly fitted harness, etc., will sometimes be the cause of peculiar actions of the horse, which might cause the inexperienced to conclude that they are sick.

You can only learn to intelligently recognize abnormal actions of the horse after you have studied the normal animal long enough to know all the peculiarities that usually belong to it.

CHAPTER X

THE VALUE OF EXERCISE AND CONDITION IN PREVENTION OF DISEASE

We hear the term "condition" used, but not always in just the right manner. By the term "condition" many people think that we are always referring to the present state of the health, but in the sense that we use it, we mean the animal's physical fitness to thoroughly perform bodily or muscular work. So when we speak of a horse being "soft" or "out of condition" or "lacking in condition," or "in the pink of condition," we are referring to two conditions, one just the opposite of the other. In the draft or work horse condition does not have the same meaning that it does for the race horse or the sporting horse as they are called upon to perform to the limit of the endurance for a short space of time, while the work of the draft horse is slow and deliberate.

With farm horses it is possible in the spring season to take sufficient time during the first work of the spring to bring about a gradual conditioning. With some classes of work, this is not possible, as it requires too much haste, so such animals must be conditioned by methodical exercising before being put to such work. Fire department horses and army artillery horses are very good examples of these.

The horse that has spent the winter in idleness and the fat sleek horses that come from the dealers

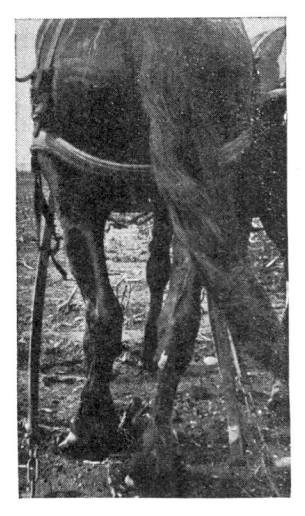

This condition is often spoken of as a "jack." It is a bone spavin. Usually makes the horse lame. *Courtesy Prof. R. S. Hudson, Michigan State College.*

are fat, soft and flabby, and are easily fatigued and exhausted. Every organ and structure in the body has been doing just the amount of work that was necessary to digest the food, carry the animal from place to place as occasion demanded, and to maintain the other bodily functions. When it is suddenly called upon to do more than this, it becomes rapidly fatigued and exhausted. The lungs must become accustomed to breathing more air, the heart to pumping the blood faster, the joints to the performing of a greater number of movements and the muscles to exert more force and more movements.

How to Obtain Condition

This can only be done by a judicious combination of good wholesome feed and plenty of exercise carried on for some little length of time. The exercise should not be forced and it should be graduated. The work should not be severe nor over such a length of time as to fatigue the animal. If overexertion is practiced, the animal will lose flesh; this is a common fault with most men in beginning their farm work in the spring of the year; they work their horses too hard. Many trainers also work their harness horses too hard. It indicates poor horsemanship to see a horse being worked when he is too tired to do his work with safety. It is a frequent cause of accidents and injuries and is to be condemned under all conditions. The ability to distinguish the fact that the muscular development is becoming more pronounced, and of keeping the amount of work within the limits of the ability of the animal is the proof of good horsemanship. As soon as a horse is in good condition or is seasoned, a fair amount of work will do him no injury at all, but will gradually add to the condition. Horses that are conditioned properly do not lose great amounts of flesh during the early working season.

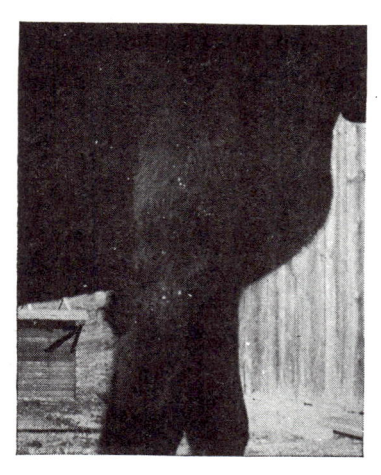

This horse has a shoe boil. Early treatment is advisable. *Courtesy Prof. R. S. Hudson, Michigan State College.*

Amount and Kind of Work

In the work horse the kind of work will vary; with the farm horse it usually consists in the preparing of the soil for the spring crops. With most farmers, there is usually several days work early in the spring that must be performed before the heavier work begins; such as breaking corn stalks, hauling manure, repairing fences, hauling of various kinds, and the like. Under these conditions, the farm horse usually has quite a little light work before the heavy work begins. But regardless of the work, the horse should not be worked until it is greatly fatigued and should be rested often. If the farmer has nothing of a light nature for the team to do, and does not live too far from his marketing center, it would be advisable to use the team hitched to the wagon for the frequent trips that he usually makes to town. This will be very good exercise and will help condition the animals, and toughen the shoulders. The exercise or work should always be at the walk and if the animals have been idle for any length of time, this will require some little patience on the part of the driver. The amount of work or exercise and the length of time should be gradually increased, at first two hours of fairly brisk walking can be increased slightly each day and the animal gradually put to light work, such as hauling light loads in the wagon, etc.

Effect of Feeding

As the exercise or work increases, the feed must be increased also. It is impossible to efficiently condition a horse on a light diet. It requires no little amount of judgment to properly ration the feed to the amount of work that the animal is doing, and the ability to do so only comes from actual experience. If the work is too hard for the amount of feed the animal is receiving, he loses his sleek glossy

THE VALUE OF EXERCISE

appearance; as we often say, he loses his "bloom" or fresh appearance.

Features of Early Training

Thirst and sweating of early training of animals are very important features and really are closely associated. The sweating of young horses is very noticeable and is many times due to nervousness. For this reason, it is always best when working the young or highly nervous animal to treat them as

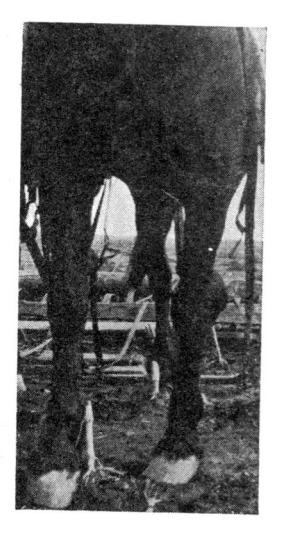

A typical case of wind gall or wind puff in the horse. Do not often cause the horse any trouble, but are unsightly. *Courtesy Prof. R. S. Hudson, Michigan State College.*

102 SOME COMMON DISEASES OF THE HORSE

quietly as possible. An experienced horseman does not tire the young horse with long, monotonous lessons, but proceeds with orderliness and concludes the lesson as soon as possible. When animals are sweating freely, they become quite thirsty. Thirsty horses may be allowed to drink as much as they want if they are moved about until they are cooled, to prevent their becoming chilled. This thirstiness will diminish as their condition improves.

The quantity and quality of the sweat is usually taken as an indication of condition. The horse that is green or soft will produce great quantities of soapy lathery sweat and will not dry very fast. As condition improves, the animal dries faster, the sweat becomes more watery and the animal requires more work to produce the sweating. Some animals sweat very easily, even when in good condition, and others due to their nervous dispositions, so these two latter factors are not to be overlooked.

The weather conditions have much to do with the cause of sweating; it requires much work on a clear, dry cold day, while horses sweat very easily on a damp, muggy, stuffy day.

CHAPTER XI

HOW TO GIVE MEDICINES TO THE HORSE

The inexperienced find it rather difficult to give medicines to the horse by the mouth. This is due to the size and strength of the horse and his lack of adaptability to strange conditions and new situations. A horse will not favor a change of any kind and when it finds itself in a new position it often loses its power of self control.

The following methods of giving medicines are commonly used: with the grain, in the drinking water, by drenching and with a dose syringe. The hypodermic syringe is largely used by veterinarians, as well as the capsule; they are not available in the ordinary stable, but the technique could very easily and quickly be learned. In some few cases medicines are given on the tongue.

Medicines may be given in the powdered form, in a watery solution or in the form of a paste. The method used in administering and the physical characteristics as well as the nature of the working of the medicine will largely determine the form in which it is given.

In respiratory cases in which the breathing is difficult, the giving of medicines by the way of the mouth as a drench is not to be recommended, owing to the danger of mechanical pneumonia due to the breathing of a portion of the liquid. As a general practice medicines that do not require great dilution to prevent irritation should not be greatly diluted as this adds to the difficulty of giving and also increases the dangers from it.

Drenching

This is by far the most common method of giving medicine to the horse, also the most dangerous from the manner in which it is ordinarily done. It is the only method that many individuals are acquainted with and for this reason is in common use. A horse should never be drenched through the nose under any conditions and while it is often done, it has killed several times as many horses as all other methods combined. Horses should only be drenched through the mouth, when drenched at all. This can best be done by taking the horse and turning it, end for end, in the stall; secure a small rope and make a small loop at one end just large enough to go over the upper jaw that will not slip tight. The loose end of the rope is then placed back of the nose band (this is to prevent the loop slipping off the upper jaw) and then over a beam or through a ring placed at the ceiling and the animal's head drawn up till it is slightly extended. This arrangement does not permit the animal getting the tongue behind the liquid

HOW TO GIVE MEDICINES

as readily as when the pressure is on the under jaw; a long necked bottle is used for the solution; the neck is inserted into one side of the mouth, just in front of the molar teeth, and a small quantity of the solution poured into the mouth. Too much solu-

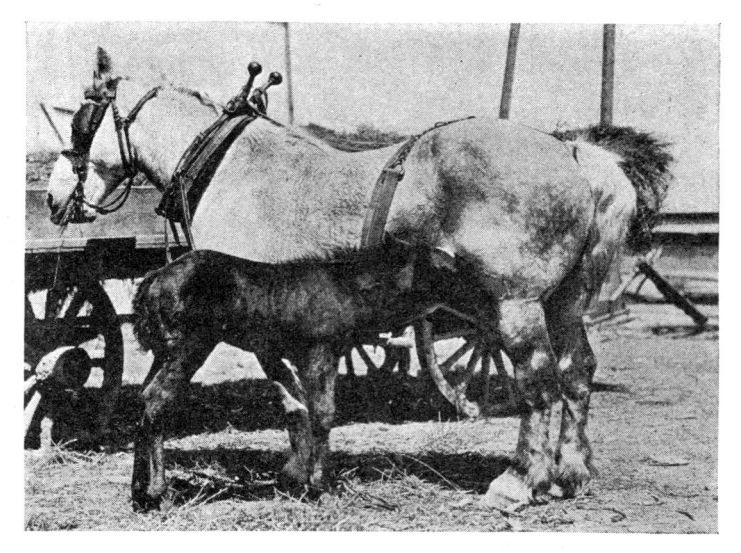

This grade percheron mare is doing her share of the farm work and doing a good job of raising her colt. *Courtesy of Prof. R. S. Hudson, Michigan State College.*

tion should not be poured into the mouth at one time, for this may produce strangulation. Care must be taken that the neck of the bottle does not become broken between the teeth. Swallowing may be induced by massaging the throat, and in obstinate cases a little clean water may be poured into one of the nostril. This should in no instance be more than a

106 SOME COMMON DISEASES OF THE HORSE

tablespoonful. If drenching is done often, it is best to have a rubber bottle for this purpose. Drenching the horse is a dirty, dangerous, hard task, and for the good of the horse and the operator as well, should only be practiced when absolutely necessary.

The Dose Syringe

This is by far the most popular method and has the advantage of being cleaner, more sure of animals getting the entire dose and saves time. Syringes are not very expensive and are commonly used in the two ounce size; they are also made in one and four ounce sizes for those who care for that size. The syringe is filled and held in the right hand in the proper position for expelling its contents; the left hand is passed between the upper and lower jaw on the right side and through the inter-dental space (this is the space in both jaws between the incisor and molar teeth) and grasps the tongue firmly from above; this finds the thumb pointing toward the incisor teeth. The hand is then rotated upward and back until the thumb rests in the roof of the mouth; this opens the animal's mouth in good position for giving the medicine. The nozzle of the syringe is inserted through the space on the left side and the contents thrown well back in the mouth. The syringe is quickly withdrawn and the tongue is released. With a little practice this is the safest, quickest and surest method of medicating the horse.

In a Capsule

These capsules are the ordinary gelatin capsule but are of much larger capacity; those used in the horse usually holding one ounce. The same pro-

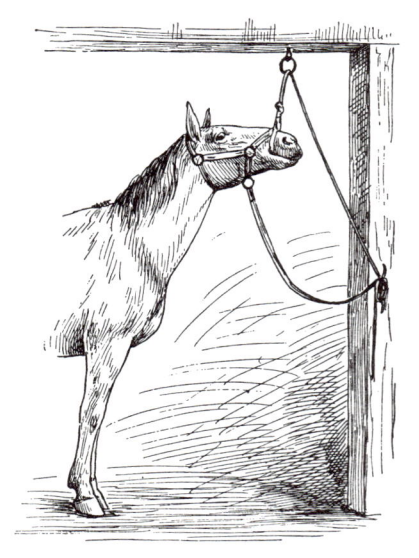

A good method for use in drenching the horse.

cedure is used in giving these as is used with the dose syringe. Special instruments called balling guns are used to place the capsule on the back of the tongue where it can be swallowed or it can be placed there by the use of the hand. A small hand is an asset in this work. The tongue is grasped and held just as though a dose syringe were being used. The capsule is held with the ends of the fingers forming a cone, the hand holding the capsule is inserted over the top of the mouth and well back in the animal's mouth with considerable haste. Too much wasted time usually results in injury to the hand on the teeth of the animal during its attempt at swallowing. In giving capsules, the operator should have one assistant who stands on the left side of the animal with his right hand on the neck or shoulder and the left hand grasping the nose in the region of the nose band; this is for the purpose of preventing the animal throwing its head up or sidewise, while the operator has his hand in the mouth. The halter should be large enough to permit the animal to open the mouth wide enough that it will not interfere with the operator. This requires quite a little practice but is not difficult to learn.

With the Grain

Medicines that do not have an objectionable odor and taste and that are not irritating in their original form are often mixed with the grain as it is fed to the animal. A very good way when it can be employed. The common practice is to feed it on bran, middlings or chop feed, preferably on bran.

In the Drinking Water

There are a few remedies that can be given in this way; the dose of medicine is placed in a pail of

HOW TO GIVE MEDICINES

drinking water. The medicine must be practically free from taste and odors, to be administered in this way.

On the Tongue

For local conditions affecting the mouth and throat, medicines are frequently made into a thick sticky paste, with powdered licorice and glycerine and placed upon the tongue with a smooth paddle or spoon. To place on the tongue, the tongue is secured as in giving medicine, with the dose syringe and drawn slightly forward to facilitate the placing of the substance upon the tongue.

In administering medicines to the horse, it is well to remember that there is no one particular method of giving medicines. That method which is quickest, easiest, safest and best under the existing conditions, is the one to use.

CHAPTER XII

GENERAL CARE OF THE SICK HORSE

In caring for a sick horse there are certain fundamentals that should be practiced; (1) the animal should be made as comfortable as can conveniently be done, (2) it should be protected against cold or inclement weather or draughts, (3) it should be fed only palatable and appetizing feed.

If the caretaker of the sick horse can recall the kind of treatment and care that he requires when he is sick and will then keep these things in mind when caring for his sick patient, he will not be so likely to do many things that are useless or that will hinder the recovery of his patient. With the sick horse, the same as with people, there are many conditions that require very little treatment, but excellent nursing. In many conditions the nursing is often of greater importance than any medicinal treatment that can be given.

The horse is more susceptible to infections than most of the other domestic animals; therefore these diseases are always very serious when affecting this class of animals. Experienced horsemen also know that these animals also become very serious when affected with intestinal conditions; colics and indigestions are always serious in the horse and often

GENERAL CARE OF THE SICK HORSE 111

fatal. The digestive system of the horse is very delicate and for this reason the patient often dies from an inflammation of the bowels (enteritis) from what appears to be a very slight attack of indigestion

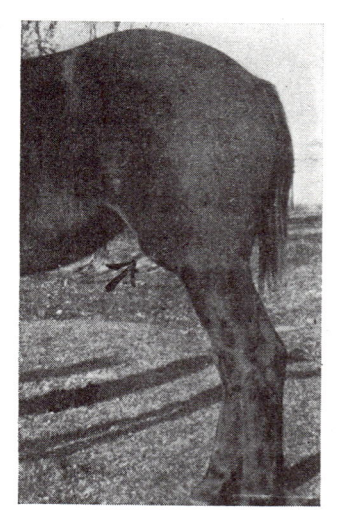

This horse is stifled. This injury is somewhat common. Should be treated early. *Courtesy Prof. R. S. Hudson, Michigan State College.*

(colic) or diarrhea, when first noticed. Because of this peculiarity, such diseases of the horse should not be neglected but should be treated promptly.

Make the Horse Comfortable

The first thing to be done when the horse is sick is to make it as comfortable as possible; place in a large, well bedded stall where the horse can lie down without any danger of becoming cast and unable to get up. A sick horse should not be kept tied in a small single stall under any conditions when sick. A temporary stall can be prepared in a few minutes' time at little or no expense. Many sick horses are lost because they are not properly stabled, but get fast in their stall and so completely exhaust themselves that treatment is of no value.

The bedding should be fresh and clean and well shaken out. Make a good, dry bed for the sick horse and keep it that way at all times. There is nothing else that I can recall now that would cause any more discomfort to the horse than a damp bed made from soiled bedding.

To increase the comfort of the sick horse, provide as much sunlight as possible; sunlight is a good tonic for the sick of any species. Unless the animal is suffering from some condition of the eyes that makes it necessary to keep the animal in the dark, provide all the sunlight that can be had.

Ventilation is very essential because the animal needs all the fresh, pure air that can be secured. This carries off the noxious odors from the discharges and assists in keeping the quarters dry and sanitary. There is no objection or danger to complete ventilation, when the patient is protected from draughts. Lack of pure, fresh air is often the cause of failure to secure recovery.

Clothing the Sick Horse

The sick horse should be well groomed and well rubbed down before being blanketed and bandaged. To keep a sick horse for several days without groom-

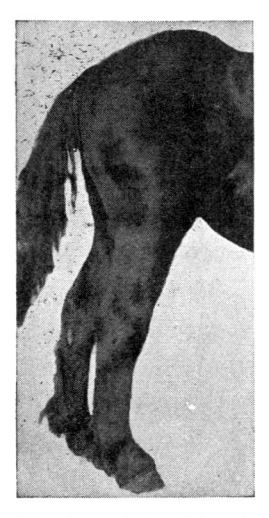

This horse's hind leg is too straight and is often spoken of as "Post Leg." Do not use such an animal for breeding. *Courtesy Prof. R. S. Hudson, Michigan State College.*

ing and bandaging the legs, is just the same as failure to bathe or wash the patient or comb its hair.

When the weather is cool the sick horse should be well blanketed; the legs should be bandaged with cotton; the bandages should be removed twice daily and the legs given a thorough massaging with the hands or a rubbing cloth, after which the bandages should be replaced. When the weather is extremely cold it may be necessary to use more than a single blanket to keep the patient warm.

In grooming the sick horse a thorough massaging with a soft brush or with rubbing cloths is desirable. If there is danger of the animal chilling, get some one to help with the grooming so that the patient need not be uncovered very long. In grooming, it is advisable to groom with the blanket turned back rather than entirely removed; this will help in preventing chilling.

During warm weather when a blanket is not needed, the use of a fly sheet will be very helpful in preventing the annoyance from flies and other insects.

Feeding and Watering

If you have ever been sick enough not to want anything to eat nor to see anything before you that you would ordinarily relish, then you know how many sick horses feel toward the feed that is placed before them. One would think from the efforts some horse owners make to force a sick animal to eat, that they thought their very life depended upon their not missing a meal. As a general thing a few meals missed by a sick horse are not going to be of much consequence, because the digestive system is

GENERAL CARE OF THE SICK HORSE

often in such a condition that it should be rested and not forced to digest feed.

As a general thing the use of such vegetables as carrots, apples, etc. will be relished by the sick horse as soon as he can be gotten to eat anything. A hot bran mash well salted will also be relished by many horses.

Do not put feed before the horse and let it remain longer than a few minutes, as it usually becomes soiled and unfit for eating; if it is not eaten in 20 to 30 minutes, it should be removed. We have seen horse owners place feed before sick horses and let it remain until the sight of it was nauseating to the horse as well as anyone that might see it.

Feed should be offered every two or three hours in very small amounts and all uneaten feed should be removed in 20 to 30 minutes. It should always be offered in clean feed boxes.

During cold weather the chill should always be removed from the drinking water. Even during summer weather, extremely cold water should not be given to the sick horse.

Special methods of feeding the sick horse are often prescribed by your veterinarian, and of course should be carried out as they direct.

During the summer months when pasture is available the sick horse will often eat grass when it can be secured; if the horse is in condition to do so, it can crop the grass or, if it cannot do this, the grass can be cut and given to it.

Another procedure that will greatly add to the comfort of the sick horse is to wash the face and nostrils two or three times each day and to rinse out the mouth. With luke warm water and a large sponge wash out the nostrils, also the secretion from the corners of the eyes; fill the sponge with water, then insert the sponge several inches inside the mouth and empty its contents by squeezing; this should be done two or three times daily.

When the horse is on the road to recovery, a laxative ration containing wheat bran and oil meal should be used to assist in keeping the bowels in good condition. It is generally best not to feed any corn at this time. A very satisfactory mixture for use when the horse is recovering, which should be mixed with the grain, is artificial Carlsbad Salt; the formula is as follows:

Dried Sodium Sulphate .... 40 parts
Sodium Bicarbonate .... 35 "
Sodium Chloride .... 15 "
Potassium Sulphate .... 2 "

One or two heaping tablespoonsful should be added to the grain ration two or three times daily. This can be continued for several days.

CHAPTER XIII

COLIC OR INDIGESTION

Both of these terms are used to indicate the fact that the animal is suffering pain in some location of the digestive tract. It is not uncommon to find many owners that think that the term indigestion has a different meaning than the word colic, and they seem to think that it is of more severity. Colic is the name given these conditions by the horseman, while the veterinarian uses the term indigestion. The latter term is to be preferred, as the word colic really means pain, and does not make any discrimination as to the origin or action of it.

Indigestions are classified according to their mode of attack and their location in the digestive tract. Thus we have congestion of the stomach, acute indigestion of the stomach, but the conditions of the bowels or intestines are usually of a sub-acute nature and we have impactions or stoppages of practically every portion of the intestines. The acute colics are more severe. The pain is greater and the rapidity with which the animal succumbs is much greater. With the conditions of the intestines, especially the large one, the animal does not evidence so much pain and the attack may persist from several hours to a few days. With acute cases of colic, it is unusual

118 SOME COMMON DISEASES OF THE HORSE

to have a case linger more than a few hours unless they show some signs of recovery.

The horse with acute colic which may be caused from an engorgement of feed in any part of the intestinal tract, or from an accumulation of gas from bloating, will show great uneasiness and pain, will get up and down at short intervals, show an anxious expression of the face, quickened breathing and in bad cases, will break out into profuse sweat. The animal cannot be kept upon its feet and will roll and make every effort to get into some position that will give it some relief. When there is bloating of the stomach, it is not unusual for the animal to sit on the haunches, just the same as a dog. If the pain is unusually severe, the animal may bite at the sides and may even roll upon its back to get relief. Horses with acute indigestion will often have periods several minutes in length, in which they show no evidence of pain. At other times, animals with indigestion are observed eating during the periods of pain. This is not an indication that the animal is improving but is the result of the agonizing pain.

Horses affected with a stoppage or an impaction of the large bowels show altogether different symptoms; they are listless and refuse to eat. Occasionally look around at the flank, may lie down and roll upon the side and lie there stretched out as if resting. He may lie this way for many minutes at a time. The bowels may move two or three times but in very small quantities. The animal may stretch out as if intending to

COLIC OR INDIGESTION

stale, and the owner will usually insist that if the animal could urinate that it would be relieved. This is brought about by the distended bowel irritating the bladder by pressing upon it. This class of cases rarely show much pain at any time. The writer has seen many cases that showed very little symptoms aside from the fact that they would not eat and had

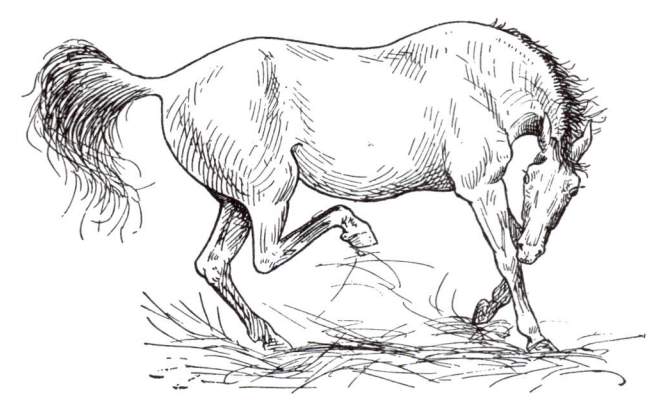

Showing how the horse usually acts with acute indigestion (colic).

no passage from the bowels. If the animal is being worked, and it has been noticed that for a short while preceding the attack the bowels have moved quite often, but in small quantities, it is well to suspect an impaction. I have known cases that have stooled as many as from five to eight times in the short period of $1\frac{1}{2}$ to 2 hours preceding the first evidence of pain. It is this class of indigestion that taxes the ability of the veterinarian and the patience of the owner. These cases will many times persist for several hours before showing any signs of a change; it is not infrequent to find them of three or four, even five days duration, and then recovering. When you consider that stasis in man of one week would be equal to that of the horse for only one day of 24 hours, you can readily understand that those cases that do not get relief for three or four days are equal to the same condition in man of from three to four weeks, and yet I have frequently seen recovery in horses after the third day. The large bulk of material usually found in the horse's intestines, accounts for the difficulty of treating this condition to get quick results. It requires many hours for liquids to soften this mass. If the continued pressure of this material upon the bowels has not paralyzed the bowel walls before this has taken place, a few doses of a quick acting cathartic will usually bring about the desired results.

These conditions can and are prevented in animals that are fed and exercised properly. Regularity of feeding has more influence upon the health of the horse than is usually thought by one who has not had an opportunity of observing the evil results from it. In the author's experience in the U. S. Army Remounts with no less than twenty-five thousand animals and covering a period of fifteen months, I feel very conservative in saying that there were not more than 25 cases of indigestion.

Feed in the proper amounts and only of good

COLIC OR INDIGESTION

quality; never feed spoiled or poor quality feed. Hay that is coarse and woody often predisposes to these conditions. When the animal is idle cut down the grain ration and enforce suitable exercise. Do not feed the animal when it is exhausted or greatly fatigued, nor when it is extremely hot. If the animal is in this condition, it should be permitted to rest before being fed. The condition of the animal's bowels should be noted carefully and kept in proper condition by the feeding of bran or linseed meal.

The first thing to do when an animal develops an attack of indigestion is to call a good veterinarian at once. It will do no hurt for you to give a quart of linseed oil, into which you have placed three or four tablespoonsful of spirits of turpentine; this is a laxative and the turpentine prevents fermentation or bloating. The next thing to do is to make the animal as comfortable as possible and allow it all the water it will drink. Water will do no hurt and you can make no mistake in allowing the animal all it will drink. Take away all feed until the doctor arrives. It is not advisable to give every manner of treatment that is said to be good in these conditions, but simply carry out the veterinarian's instructions, and usually the better results will be obtained.

The following is a very good stock mixture to have in the stable at all times, so that you will have a treatment to use if your veterinarian cannot be secured:

    Chloral hydrate .... 1 ounce
    Spirits of turpentine .... 1 ounce

Ether U.S.P. .... 1 ounce
Salicylic acid .... 3 drams
Oil of peppermint .... 2 drams
Fluid Extract of capsicum .... 1 dram
Grain alcohol to make 8 ounces

Give one (1) ounce and repeat in 1 hour if needed. Call your veterinarian promptly.

Impaction or Stoppage of the Bowels

This condition is very common during the winter months, and especially among horses that are being fed coarse woody feeds and are not getting sufficient exercise. The impaction may occur in most any location of the intestinal tract, but it is much more common in the large bowels, occurring particularly in a short loop located near the pelvis.

Such conditions as incomplete or complete twist of the bowels, slipping of one portion of the bowel within its own walls, or a strangulated hernia, which will frequently occur in stallions, should not be discussed here.

The nature of the large intestines of the horse and the large amounts of coarse indigestible feed they are called upon to handle, explains the cause for many causes of this kind. The age of the animal as well as the condition of its teeth will have considerable bearing on the occurrence of this condition. The short time that the feed has to remain in the digestive tract, and the temperament of the animal, all have a

COLIC OR INDIGESTION

bearing on this condition. It hardly seems that heredity would have any bearing on such diseases but we know that horses whose sire or dam have been often affected with digestive troubles, often are affected themselves.

The feeding and watering of the horse has by far the greatest influence upon the number of cases of this kind that occur, irregular feeding, overfeeding, change of manner of watering, allowing water when tired, overworking, the eating of indigestible materials, such as sand and dead grass. All in all, by far the greatest number of cases are the result of faulty feeding.

The symptoms of such cases are never exactly the same in any two cases, but as a general rule, the difference is largely a matter of degree rather than of kind, and is accounted for from the variation in the attack. The usual symptoms are dull pains, which will in many cases occasion no alarm, unless the owner has had previous experience with this condition. The animal eats and drinks little or nothing and after a time will walk about slowly, if loose, smelling at the bedding or the ground, and will occasionally paw with its front feet or stamp with its hind ones. It will crouch as if to lie down but will usually not do so until it has made several attempts. The horse will usually lie flat on the side for long periods of time, raising its head from time to time to look back at its side. It will hold the breath and will release it with a moan or a grunt.

124 SOME COMMON DISEASES OF THE HORSE

The above symptoms may last for several hours but after 24 to 36 hours, if improvement is not taking place, a different type of symptoms usually begin to show up. The animal shows much more pain and will lie down and get up almost continually. It has an anxious expression and the legs and ears are cold. A cold sweat breaks out under the belly and between the fore and hind legs. The animal will throw itself down violently on the ground or floor, much as if being shot or stunned by a hard blow. Cases showing such symptoms usually die in a short time.

Such conditions should be prevented by regularity in feeding, watering and exercising and good feed of a laxative nature and of good quality should be given when the animal is idle just the same as when it is at work. A good veterinarian should always be called but a quart of raw linseed oil in which three or four tablespoonsful of turpentine has been mixed is excellent and will do much good. If no veterinarian is to be had, the following will do very well:

Ammonium carbonate or muriate . . 4 ounces
Powd. nux vomica . . . . ½ ounce
Powd. ginger . . . . 1 ounce
Capsicum . . . . 1 dram

Mix well and of this give a level tablespoonful to adult horses, diluted in water or milk, every two hours. For one or two year olds, give one tablespoonful. This should be well diluted.

Diarrhea or Scours

This condition is often found in some driving horses or even in work horses that are worked faster than a walk and such horses are known as being "washy." They are usually flat sided horses with a tucked up abdomen.

Diarrhea is nature's effort to remove some offending material from the digestive tract. This offending material may be caused by feeding irregularly, by feeding when overheated or by indigestible feed or by sudden change in feed. Mistakes in feeding are responsible for most of these conditions. It must be kept in mind that the horse is a creature of habit and under no conditions should sudden changes in feeding and watering be made.

The symptoms are few but always recognizable, the passing of watery stools at frequent intervals. This gradually develops an offensive odor and will in time cause considerable irritation.

It is not advisable to stop diarrhea too suddenly and usually a mild laxative should be given. Two ounces of castor oil or one pint of raw linseed oil or even a drench of ground slippery elm bark can be given. Proper attention to feeding and watering will prevent most of such trouble. For horses that scour on the road one or two tablespoonsful of chalk with the grain ration daily will have a tendency to correct this trouble.

One of the best diarrhea remedies that we have used is the following:

Ferrous sulphate ....1 ounce
Tannic acid ....1 ounce
Sodium salicylate ....2 ounces

Give one or two tablespoonsful in water three or four times per day.

CHAPTER XIV

DISEASES OF THE BREATHING SYSTEM

Cold in the Head (Catarrh)

This condition is one of the most common affecting horses and usually in the acute form. It is then spoken of as a cold and ordinarily needs little save careful dieting and good care. Occasionally this develops into a chronic condition which is often very aggravating to handle.

The usual symptoms in acute catarrh is a watery discharge from the nose and eyes, which often becomes heavy and sticky as the disease progresses. It sometimes has a foul odor. The membranes lining the nose and eyes are inflamed. The animal rattles or snuffles as it breathes, which is faster than normal.

Due to infection and involvement of the sinus and the turbinated bones in the head, this condition often becomes chronic. A discharge will be noticed coming from the nostrils more or less continually and the animal will usually be thin and out of condition.

Acute cases should be kept in dry, warm, well ventilated quarters. Should have only good wholesome

128 SOME COMMON DISEASES OF THE HORSE

feed of a laxative nature. Little or no medical attention is needed, but a tablespoonful of saltpeter added to the drinking water once daily will be of some help.

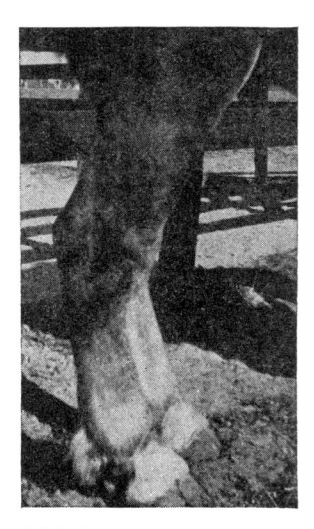

This horse shows what is spoken of as a set hock. Do not use such animals for breeding purposes. *Courtesy Prof. R. S. Hudson, Michigan State College.*

Chronic cases are much more difficult to handle and results are many times unsatisfactory. A veterinarian is usually required. A good digestive tonic is of value. The following is a good one:

Powdered nux vomica : . . . . 3 ounces
Powdered gentian . . . . 4 ounces

Powdered ginger .... 4 ounces
Sodium bicarbonate .... 6 ounces

Of this give one tablespoonful at each meal.

Bronchitis

This condition is an inflammation of the large branches of the windpipe and is usually found associated with other breathing diseases.

It is caused by exposure to damp weather when overheated or out of condition, to the breathing of smoke or other irritants and often follows colds.

The first thing noticed is usually a chill, which is closely followed by a very high fever which may reach 105 to 106 degrees F. The breathing is very fast but does not seem to give the animal much pain. At first there is a dry husky cough which changes to a moist cough. The animal often coughs up considerable mucus. The appetite is poor or altogether absent and the animal is constipated. If the ear is placed over the region of the windpipe near the chest a whistling sound will be heard. The urine is scanty and usually dark colored. Many horses do not lie down during an attack.

Good feeding and care are of most value in handling such cases. Give stimulants in early stages and a quart of very strong black coffee in which two or three tablespoonsful of aromatic spirits of ammonia has been placed is good. Laxatives such as raw linseed oil and laxative feeds should be given. Do not give aloes as it is too severe. Allow all the water the animal will drink. A mustard plaster placed over the lungs covered with a paper and blanket are excellent. Bandage the animal's legs and massage them well night and morning after removing the bandages.

The following makes a very excellent remedy for the cough:

    Ammonium muriate .... ½ ounce
    Fluid extract belladonna .... ½ ounce
    Fluid extract of nux vomica ...... 1 ounce
    Simple syrup to make 8 ounces

Of this preparation give 1 tablespoonful three or four times per day.

Congestion of the Lungs

This is an engorgement of the lungs with blood and often occurs during the winter season in fat horses that do not have sufficient exercise.

The horse breathes hard, sweats very freely and turns his head to his side. There is an anxious expression and the muscles tremble. The breathing is labored and fast. The nostrils are greatly dilated and the mucous membranes of the nose and eyes are congested and inflamed.

If the animal is stopped early and well blanketed, the legs rubbed briskly and a cold compress applied over the lungs the condition rapidly subsides. Give aromatic spirits of ammonia in 1 ounce doses well di-

DISEASES OF THE BREATHING SYSTEM 131

luted with water every three or four hours after the acute symptoms have passed. If congestion persists for any length of time apply a mustard plaster. This condition should have the best of attention for it often develops into pneumonia. Get your veterinarian at once.

Pneumonia or Lung Fever

This condition is known by four different prefixes such as "lobar," "bronchial," "pleura" and "catarrhal pneumonia" which indicates the nature of the condition. For all practical purposes the term pneumonia is sufficient.

Exposure to wet and inclement weather, overexertion, may follow a cold, also caused by irritating fumes such as smoke, drenching through the nostrils.

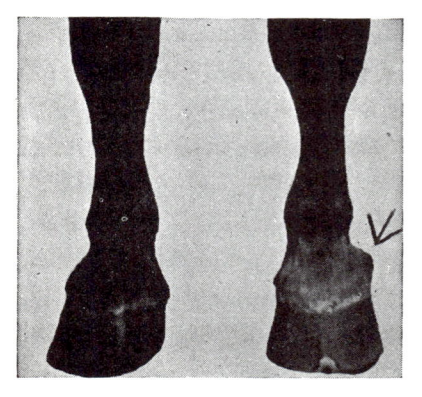

This is a sidebone. Usually produces lameness which is often incurable. *Courtesy Prof. R. S. Hudson, Michigan State College.*

Damp, cold and crowded stables all predispose to this condition. The disease itself is caused by a germ, but the above are all predisposing conditions which make the animal susceptible to it. This disease starts very similar to congestion of the lungs and in most cases this is the first stage. The animal stands with its head down and with drooping ears. Most animals remain on their feet through an attack or until they are completely exhausted. The appetite is lost and the animal is constipated. A harsh grating whistling sound is heard when the ear is placed over the lungs. If the animal has pleurisy with this, which is an inflammation of the lining of the chest cavity, a distinct ridge will be noticed extending from the region of the flank down to the lower end of the ribs.

Horses affected with pneumonia like fresh air and nothing is better for them than this, if there are no draughts.

Pneumonia reaches the climax at about the sixth day at which time the temperature reaches the highest point. Very little medication is to be recommended, save careful nursing and stimulants and good dieting to conserve the patient's strength. The animal should be covered with a good warm blanket, placed in a dry, well ventilated box stall, the legs rubbed well two or three times daily and then bandaged.

Many times the horse is not noticed when it is having the chill which is often the first symptom. If

DISEASES OF THE BREATHING SYSTEM

it is observed treat as congestion of the lungs. A veterinarian should prescribe treatment as soon as one can be secured. After the chill has subsided it is helpful to place a tablespoonful of saltpeter in the drinking water once each day.

Early in the attack a mustard plaster should be applied by mixing ground mustard seed in warm water making a paste fairly thin which should then be plastered over the chest walls working it into the hair, after which it should be covered with an oil cloth or a piece of canvas, which is in turn covered with a blanket. When it has served its purpose it can be brushed out of the hair.

Remember good care and careful feeding are of more value in pneumonia than any medicinal treatment. Complete recovery rarely takes place in less than three weeks.

Heaves

Heaves is a chronic disease of the breathing organs, that has resulted from chronic dilation or rupture of the air sacs in the lungs.

Contrary to the usual belief this disease is not caused by eating dusty or spoiled hay or feed, but is caused by over-loading the stomach, which presses on the large nerve that supplies the lungs, with the result that the small air spaces lose their usual elasticity and hence the forced effort to remove the air from the lungs. This condition is often brought

134 SOME COMMON DISEASES OF THE HORSE

about by working a horse at too fast a gait when on a full stomach.

Every one at all familiar with horses has observed the peculiar double expiratory effort of a horse with heaves. This breathing is most pronounced when the animal is exercised on a full stomach. Usually there is a moist grunting cough, the nostrils are dilated and occasionally mucous is passed from the nose. The dilation of the nostrils is constant and if this is observed one need never buy a plugged horse that has heaves.

The only treatment in most cases consists of careful feeding and right kind of exercise. Give easily digested and the best of feed and do not give the animal an opportunity to gorge itself. Would advise one or two tablespoonsful of chalk with the feed night and morning.

Use Fowler's solution of arsenic as follows: begin with one teaspoonful on the feed three times per day and gradually increase until the animal is getting one tablespoonful three times each day. Keep this up for six or eight weeks or until the eyes appear puffy and watering. Discontinue then for a few days and begin as before.

CHAPTER XV

DISEASES OF THE FEET AND LEGS

Soundness is that physical ability of an animal that enables it to perform the ordinary work required of animals of its class and type; an unsoundness then is anything that will prevent an animal from the performance of those duties usually performed by it. Ringbones, side-bones, spavins, etc., are all common unsoundnesses. Most of the unsoundnesses of horses are acquired, but a few of them may be the result inherited from the parents' weaknesses.

A blemish is anything that detracts from or mars the beauty of appearance of the horse. It may or may not interfere with its usefulness; if it does it then becomes an unsoundness. There are several conditions that may fall under both classes, such as spavins, ringbones, curbs, etc. The most common blemishes are capped hocks, capped elbows, curbs, splints, puffs or wind-galls, baggy or coarse hocks, etc. It is well to keep in mind that the two terms are used interchangeably as far as conditions upon the legs are concerned. Our reason for using these terms interchangeably with spavins, ringbones, etc., is simply this. Due to structural changes that may occur in the part due to the inflammation during the course of the diseased condition, changes may be brought about that will eliminate the interference to the animal's usefulness; in the case of the spavin, the bone cells multiply very rapidly and produce a large bony growth in the region of the hock, and which become

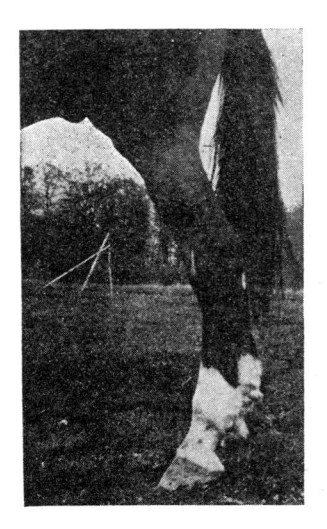

This horse is entirely too long in the gaskin (between the stifle and hock) and is therefore an undesirable type. *Courtesy Prof. R. S. Hudson, Michigan State College.*

large enough to include the entire joint, thus rendering it immovable. This enables the animal to travel without lameness, and this condition is known as anchylosis, which is simply the process of making the joint immovable. In joints in which there was extreme flexion this would interfere with

DISEASES OF FEET AND LEGS

the locomotion, but not so with the hock joint. This bony growth that we call a "spavin" is technically known as an exostosis. Splints, spavins, ringbones, are all in this class. They derive their name from their location.

Ligaments and tendons are differentiated in this way: Ligaments unite bone to bone, while tendons unite muscles to bone. The suspensory ligament, which is found upon the back part of the leg, where it passes over the fetlock joint, is the ligament that is most commonly injured.

Sweeney or Atrophy of the Shoulders

This is nothing more nor less than a wasting away or a shrinking of the muscles of the shoulder that cover the shoulder blade, caused by an injury to the nerve supplying these muscles, usually the result of side draft or an improperly fitted collar.

Capped Elbow

This is an enlargement of the tissues covering and surrounding the elbow joint, caused from bruises from the floor, but more often bruises from the heel of the shoe; also known as shoe boils; sometimes becomes quite large, but does not cause lameness. May contain serum which, if it becomes infected, will result in an abscess.

Splint

This is a bony growth on the inner side of the cannon bone, just below the knee, known as high or low splint, according to whether it is close to the joint or farther away. They do not often cause lameness but when they do, it is usually persistent and the animal will not warm out of it. As this condition is the result of the tearing of a very small ligament that holds the long splint bone to the cannon bone, splints do not occur after the animal is six years of age, as by this age their bones have united firmly, thus obliterating this ligament. Splints occurring quite near the joint frequently produce lameness in the animal. If a small pea-like enlargement is found upon both front legs where a splint normally occurs, it is well to suspect these as being natural to the horse.

Ringbones

They are the result of some irritation to the part and are found upon the small bones of the feet anywhere from the fetlock joint to the top of the hoof. A ringbone consists of a circular bony growth upon the body of one of the small bones of the foot. The size of the growth is exceedingly variable, being so small as to be hardly felt in some horses, and in others forming a large heavy ridge beneath the skin that can be seen for several feet. They are called "high ringbones" when they are near the fetlock

DISEASES OF FEET AND LEGS

joint and "low ringbones" when they are near the hoof. The low ringbone usually causes the more pronounced lameness. They are quite common in work horses and while it is not often that they ren-

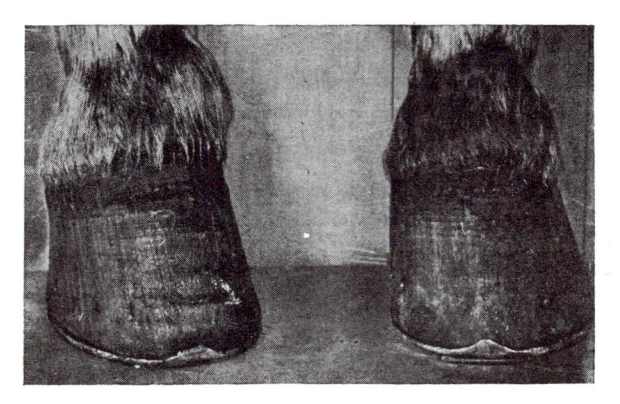

This horse had a very large ringbone as shown by the enlargements just above the hoof.

der the horse useless for work, yet they frequently cause very pronounced lameness when the animal is worked upon hard roads or pavements. Ringbones occur in all four feet.

Sidebones

They, too, are frequently found in work horses, and are simply an ossification or turning to bone of the lateral cartilage of the foot. In the normal foot, just a little in front of the heel, and just a little back of the center of the foot, you can feel with the finger a small projection that extends just above the edge of the hoof under the skin. This is the lateral cartilage and will yield upon pressure. When from some irritation this turns to bone, due to the inflammatory processes, we then speak of it as sidebone. It occurs in any of the feet and often produces very pronounced lameness in animals that are worked upon hard surfaced roads. They are most common in the front feet, but it is not an impossibility to find them in hind feet.

Sand Cracks or Hoof Cracks

This condition is also known as quarter cracks. It is the result of the excessive dryness of the horn of the hoof, which permits them to crack open, due to the pressure and concussion. This condition is not often found in animals that have their feet kept moist, nor in animals that work upon soft roads. It is simply a crack in the wall of the hoof extending down from the top toward the sole, found in the region of the toe and at the quarter. Quarter cracks are often caused by increasing the pressure in this region of the hoof from cutting away too much of the heel, when fitting the shoes. They may occur in any of the feet, and are exceedingly troublesome to handle. As a general thing, it makes the animal very lame.

Corns

They are located in the heel just under the heel of the shoe; may occur in all feet, but are commonly found only in front. It is a bruise of the sensitive part of the foot and when pressure is placed upon them, it produces lameness. If an animal has corns, the shoe should bear no weight over the corn, and if the region is struck lightly, the animal will flinch. The lameness can be eliminated by the removal of the pressure, but a horse that is affected with corns will give more or less trouble and is undesirable for a work animal.

Foundered Hoof

In horses that have been severely affected with founder or laminitis, it is not uncommon to find the toe turning up when the animal walks. The walls of the hoof contain heavy irregular rings and the sole of the foot is convex or has dropped down. This ribbed condition of the hoof should not be confused with the normal rings that occur in some horses that have been long on grass and that are known as grass rings.

Thrush

Is an affection of the frog of the foot and is no doubt due to an infection of some kind. It is characterized by a dark, tarry discharge and a very foul odor. In ordinary cases, it does not harm but in aggravated cases, it produces lameness. Owing to the difficulty of keeping the bottom of the feet dry, it is frequently difficult to receive good results during the treatment of this condition. Found in all four feet.

142   SOME COMMON DISEASES OF THE HORSE

Thoroughpin

Is a soft doughy swelling that appears in the region between the tendon and the bone and just above the hock; this can be pushed back and forth and is a protrusion of the capsular ligament between the tendons in this region. This enlargement usually ranges in size from that of a small walnut to a small hen's egg. Does not make the animal lame.

Bog Spavin

Is very similar to thoroughpin and is caused in the same way, but it occurs on the inner front side of the

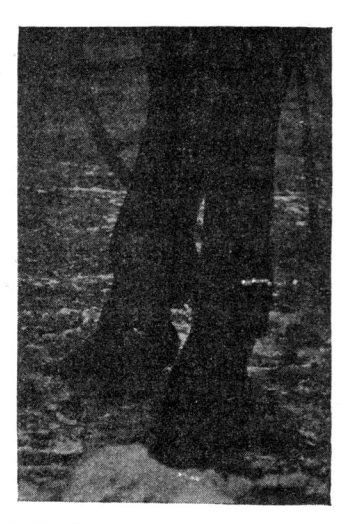

This horse is knuckling over in the hind ankle joints—this is known as cocked-ankle.

DISEASES OF FEET AND LEGS 143

hock and occurs in the depressions normally found between the tendons in this region and the bones. The greatest objection is the appearance, and the fact that it indicates more or less weakness of the hock. This enlargement is filled with the joint oil, as is that of the thoroughpin. There is frequently an enlargement on the inner side of the hock that is associated with the large vein that passes across the inner side of the hock. This is commonly referred to as a blood spavin, but it is not an unsoundness.

Bone Spavin

This is a bony growth on the inner side of the hock and varies greatly in size. It is the worst unsoundness of the horse. This can usually be detected by standing in front of the horse and observing the two hocks. It is well to remember that it is very possible to have a spavin on each hock, so it becomes necessary to understand the structure of the hock to determine this. In some cases there is not an external bony growth for some little time. These are known as "occult spavins" which means "hidden spavins." The bone spavin varies greatly in size and in some cases involves the whole inner surface of the hock and may eliminate the lameness by uniting the joint. This form of spavin usually causes lameness at some stage of its development.

Curb

It occurs only on the hind legs and just below the hock and on the large tendon that passes down the back part of the leg. It is the result of a sprain of the ligament or a rupture, of some of the fibres that compose it. It is characterized by a thickness of the ligaments, and is a variation from the straightline which should extend from the point of the hock to the fetlock joint.

The Care of the Horse's Feet

There is an old, old saying "no foot, no horse," that we quote again to impress upon you the importance of the proper treatment and care of the horse's feet. There is no part of the animal's body that requires as much attention and receives as little as does the foot of the horse. It is a well known fact that many, if not most of the unsoundnesses of the feet are the result of neglect of the animal's feet, and that they could be prevented by the use of a little care and judgment.

Under nature's own condition, the horses' feet would not be subject to such predisposing causes to injury and disease, as they are under domestication. The original plan for the horse was his gathering of his feed as he required from the native pastures and in this way the ground furnished not only a soft carpet upon which he moved about but the dew and rain soaked vegetation furnished moisture for his

DISEASES OF FEET AND LEGS 145

feet and kept them in good condition. The domestication of the horse by man changed all this and the altered conditions under which he was kept and used made him quite susceptible to diseased conditions of the feet. The use of the horse upon hot, dusty roads and upon hard slippery pavements is in conflict to the natural footing that he was to walk upon. The adoption of some protection to the foot became necessary and as permanence was desired, the iron shoe was designed; this further increased the liabilities to the feet in the way of injuries and disease. Another common cause of injury is the concussion that is produced while working on the hard surfaced roads.

According to Prof. John W. Adams, "The foot of the horse will grow from $\frac{1}{6}$ to $\frac{1}{2}$ inch per month, with a general average of about $\frac{1}{3}$ inch; unshod animals' feet will grow faster than those that are shod; the feet of geldings and mares grow faster than those of the stallions. From these statements, the necessity for giving the feet proper attention can very readily be realized.

The wall of the foot grows downward below the sole of the foot unless it is removed or becomes broken off. We have frequently seen this shell, one inch or more in length; as a usual thing, such shells are permitted to grow until they shorten themselves by breaking off at the level of the bottom of the sole. When they break in this manner, it is not unusual for them to break away more at one location of the foot than at another. In this way, the foot is not kept level and the bones that are found in the foot maintain their normal position and there will be a strain upon some of the ligaments and tendons and a relaxation of some of the others. To the horseman who has had a wide experience with horses, it is generally

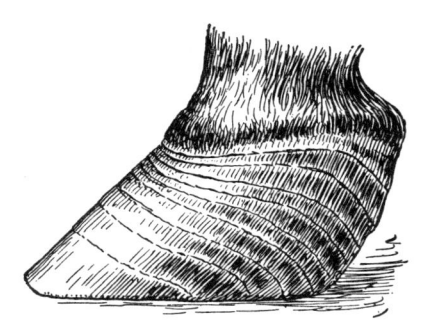

This shows the usual deformity of the foot of a horse that has been foundered (laminitis).

conceded that the throwing out of balance of the structures within the foot is no doubt the cause of by far the greatest percentage of lamenesses. In neglected feet of colts, it is not uncommon to find large flat deformed feet, or feet with wings at the quarters, etc. It is absolutely necessary to trim the colt's feet often if the desirable type of foot is to be obtained. While the toes of the foot grow faster than the heels, they also wear away faster. When the animal is shod, the wearing off of the toe is prevented and the greater amount of horn that is removed from the toe than from the heel emphasizes this fact very plainly.

DISEASES OF FEET AND LEGS

However, if the horse is to go barefoot, it should have plenty of horn, but it should not extend below the level of the bottom of the sole, or it may become broken or split from coming into contact with hard objects. The frog should be pared level (or almost so) with the sole of the foot; some of the older horseshoers are very prejudiced against cutting any of the frog away, but it does no particular damage when done within reason. The edge of the wall should be well rounded off. A horse that has been wearing shoes will not stand as much neglect as one who has always gone barefoot. Horses that are going barefoot should have their feet inspected often to detect any faults or irregularities in their growth.

At the present age, it is almost a necessity to have all work horses shod, due to the fact that the greater per cent of our roads are hard surface roads, and even the farmers' horses are frequently used upon them. Such roads are very wearing on the unshod hoof and will soon produce lameness. Even where the horse is to be used upon the farm exclusively, it is no doubt advisable to keep them shod, otherwise their feet will be neglected and undesirable growth will result with its accompanied lameness or faulty gait.

During the hot summer months or when an animal is worked upon a hard surfaced road or a pavement, it is a very common occurrence for their hoofs to become very dry and hard. This is due to the evaporation of the natural moisture of the horn. We have had cases under our care that have developed lameness at several times from this neglect. We prescribed a method of caring for the feet that would counteract this condition and as long as the owner carried out instructions, the horse went sound. This will occur most frequently with those animals that have a badly contracted heel or a badly pinched hoof head. (The hoof head is the top of the hoof where it joins the skin). The extreme dryness and hardness prevents any elasticity of the walls and pinches the delicate structures very much the same as a hard dry, stiff boot or shoe would pinch the foot. There are several hoof ointments and preparations upon the market but they are of little value unless the hoof has first been well saturated with moisture. This can be done in a number of ways—it can be done by standing the horse in cold water for two or three hours, many stables have a soaking tub or tank built in the stall for this very purpose; the water need not extend more than one or two inches above the top of the horn. It can also be accomplished very well by standing the horse in a puddle or small stream if one happens to be near. A very easy way and one that can be applied any place, is to secure large pieces of cloth and soak them in cold water and tie them around the pastern and allow them to hang over the top of the hoof. They should be wetted often. As soon as the horn has taken up sufficient moisture, its evaporation can be prevented by the use of oil or by the use of a good hoof dressing. Linseed oil or cottonseed oil, applied with a swab or a brush, will do very well. This should be applied at least once a day. A very good hoof dressing and one that improves the appearance of the horse's hoof is made as follows:

>   Pine tar .... 3 pints
>   Spirits of turpentine .... 1 pint
>   Linseed oil .... ½ gallon

Mix well and apply to the surface of the hoof with a brush. If the horse is to be taken into the dust, it is well to apply as long before going to work as possible. After the hoof is in good condition, it can be kept that way by the use of any of the methods described above.

Treatment of Conditions Affecting the Feet and Legs

Most of these conditions will respond to a general line of treatment and for that reason we give a general line of treatment. In acute cases where there is swelling and soreness such as curbs, etc., we recommend the following liniment, which should be thoroughly rubbed in three or four times daily until all swelling or pain has ceased:

>   Tincture of Aconite Root........4 ounces
>   Fluid Extract of Belladonna......4 ounces
>   Soap liniment .... 4 ounces
>   Grain alcohol ....4 ounces

For spavins, ringbones, sidebones, bowed tendons,

150 SOME COMMON DISEASES OF THE HORSE

etc., two methods of treatment can be used: A blister or an absorbent liniment. A good blister can be made as follows. Never blister an acute condition.

Red iodide of mercury .... 2 drams
Potassium iodide .... 2 drams
Glycerine .... 1 ounce
Alcohol .... 1 ounce

Apply and rub in well and if blistering is not sufficient, it can be repeated. After blistering is completed, wash blistered area with warm water and soap and grease with oil or vaseline.

A satisfactory absorbent liniment is as follows:

Oil of wormwood .... 1 ounce
Oil of turpentine .... 4 ounces
Oil of wintergreen (artificial) ... 2 ounces
Oil of mustard .... ½ ounce
Alcohol .... 8 ounces

Apply twice daily, rubbing in well but gently.

For Thrush we have found nothing better than the following:

Calomel .... 2 ounces
Iodoform .... 2 ounces
Boracic acid .... 4 ounces

Remove all the secretion from the cleft of the frog and the feather edges and then work small quantities of this powder into the bottom of the cleft with something blunt and then pack with cotton or oakum to keep the powder in and the moisture out. Keep the feet as dry as possible.

CHAPTER XVI

CONTAGIOUS DISEASES

Influenza

This condition is also spoken of as "pink eye," "typhoid fever," "gripp," which are the common names usually given to it. It is an acute infectious disease in which there is fever present. In some animals we have only a slight catarrh of the mucous membranes, while in others there is a severe inflammation of the lungs and the pleura which lines the lung cavity; the first is known as catarrhal and the latter as pectoral influenza.

This disease is very prevalent in all parts of the world and occurs in the form of an epidemic, at which time it will affect nearly all the animals in quite extensive areas. It spreads very rapidly and at times produces a very heavy loss. Many of the cases develop a fatal pneumonia, which makes this a very dangerous disease.

The cause is an infection but up until this time the primary cause of the disease has not been determined; there are two germs that are so closely associated that it has not been determined to which one the credit should belong; they are the streptococcus equi and the bacillus equisepticus.

The infection is carried from one animal to another by the secretions from the lungs and by the feces. This infection is very well marked during the height of the disease and also during convalescence. Animals that have unhealed lesions in the lungs can no doubt spread the infection for many months. The horse markets are the greatest source of this disease. It is also possible for the infection to be carried by attendants and upon stable utensils, clothing, and harness; it will also live for some little time in dark, damp, poorly ventilated stables.

The infection gains access to the animal's body through the feed and water. It may be possible that the animal may secure the infection through the lungs in some cases. This is a disease of horses of almost any age, but animals under one year of age and very old animals are not so often affected. Exposure and sudden changes in the weather, in fact anything that would tend to produce a cold or any irregularity in the normal condition of the breathing system, will predispose to this condition. An attack of the disease diminishes the animal's susceptibility for only a short time.

After the infection has gained access to the animal's body, it is usually from three to seven days before the disease is well established; in exceptional cases it may be as long as eight or nine days. If the animal has a cold the first symptoms of the disease may be noticed within 48 hours.

The first symptoms of the disease are a marked depression or listlessness and an increased appetite. The animal a little later stands with eyes closed, drooping ears and low hanging head. They may stand in very unnatural positions at this stage. The appetite begins to fail. At this stage a mouth full of feed may be chewed up and allowed to lie inside the

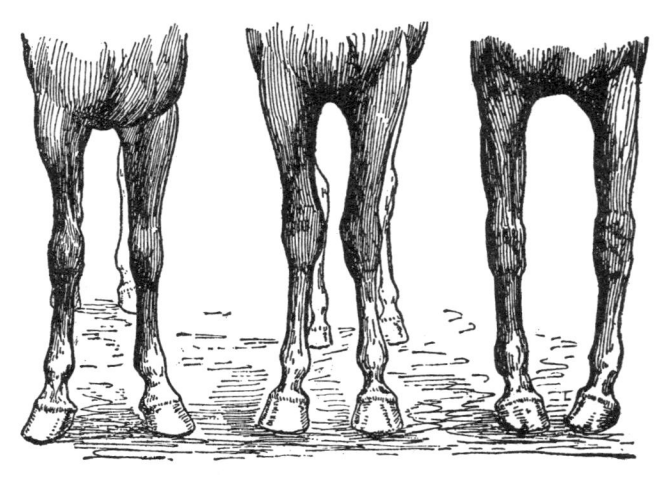

This shows 3 common faulty conformations of the front legs of the horse.

cheeks alongside the molar teeth. The animals do not move around unless urged to do so and often they do so with a weak staggering gait. The temperature goes very high and 106° F. is not at all uncommon. If it is the simple catarrhal form, it will remain at this height for two or three days and then gradually return to normal; in such cases, it will usually be around normal in from five to seven days.

If the pectoral or pneumonia form develops, the temperature will remain high and will not be lowered. The heart beat in the simple form is usually found to be from 50 to 60 per minute, while in extremely severe cases it may be from 80 to 100 per minute. The coat is rough and muscular trembling may be noticed.

In the catarrhal form we have the inflammation of the lining or conjunctivae of the eye; it becomes very red (this is the reason for calling it "pink eye") and a profuse flow of tears, which are frequently mixed with pus overflows the eye and down the side of the face. In a short while a watery discharge is noticed from the nostrils. At first a dry harsh cough is noticed but this later develops into a moist one, but it is usually strong and often gives the animal considerable pain. The glands around the jaw and throat are often slightly swollen and tender to the touch; the breathing is much faster than normal and as a rule shallow. There may be noticed at this time slight digestive disturbances, which usually become more noticeable in three or four days by the passing of very foul smelling feces. The urine is scant and very dark in color. It is not uncommon to find large swellings on the abdomen and chest and also of the sheath of geldings and stallions. The legs frequently fill up considerably.

The first symptoms of the pectoral or pneumonia form are the same as those for the catarrhal form; after two or three days they become more severe and the development of an affection of the lungs is noticed. This form is differentiated from the other form by the continued high fever, more difficult breathing which is usually of an abdominal type, sensitiveness of the chest, and often a rust colored discharge from the nostrils. If this discharge turns greenish in color and has a distinct putrefactive odor, it is an indication that gangrene of the lungs has developed; it is always fatal. Horses with this pneumonia rarely, if ever, lay down during the course of the disease.

There are many complications that may develop with this disease that makes it a very dangerous one; an inflammation of the tendons and the surrounding structures; the development of founder or laminitis; an inflammation of the bowels, blood-poisoning and hemorrhages of the lungs. Any of these complications may produce death very rapidly in an otherwise simple case of the disease.

This disease is very variable in the duration of its course, which is due, no doubt to the resistance of the animal, the manner of treatment and care that it receives and the virulence of the infection. In some cases it may terminate in two or three days, but the common length of the disease is about one week; in a few instances a week or ten days may see the end of the fever. It frequently is weeks before the animal entirely recovers. The termination of this form depends largely upon those conditions mentioned above.

This disease can very easily be mistaken for other conditions; especially is this true if there are no other outbreaks in the community. It may be confused with an ordinary form of pneumonia.

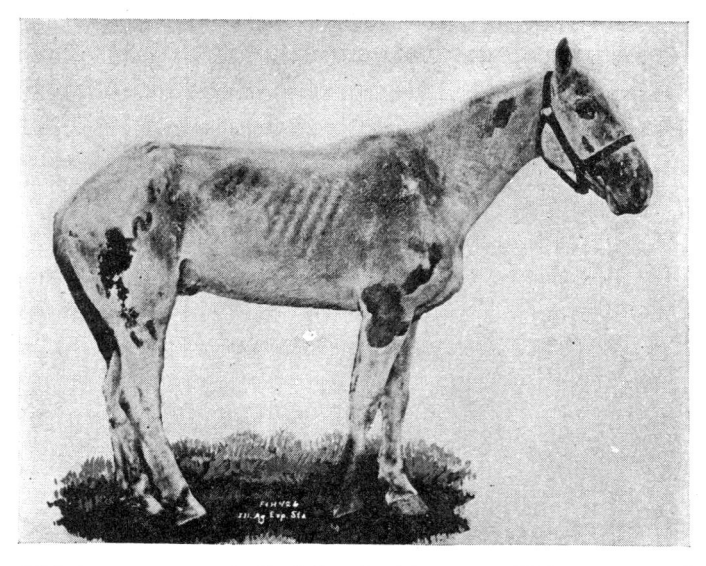

This horse was very badly infested with worms. This was an aged gelding, but even young horses are badly injured when heavily infested with worms. *Photo Illinois Agricultural Experiment Station.*

However, the spread of it to other animals in the stable and the later development of some of the characteristic symptoms will serve to differentiate it. When the disease is in the community or when it has been in the stable previously, it is well to suspect all conditions of this nature that show a temperature as being **influenza**.

CONTAGIOUS DISEASES

The losses from this disease, especially of the catarrhal form, are very light when there are no complications, and when the animals receive good care; it depends largely on the physical condition of the animal when it contracts the disease, the care it receives and the virulence or strength of the infection. Many more animals die with the pneumonia form. If the fever is not too high and the animal retains a good appetite the prospects for recovery are good. In those cases where the fever will be irregular and when it lasts more than a week, with possibly a rise, it is a very unfavorable indication. Severe inflammation of the tendons of the legs and a persistent diarrhea are both unfavorable signs.

As soon as the condition is recognized, the sick animals should be isolated from the well ones. The sick ones should be at once placed in a cool, airy, well-ventilated stall, that is well bedded and made as comfortable as possible. The food should be easily digested, palatable and, if possible, green. The animal should have plenty of pure cold water. Good care and careful feeding do as much good as anything in simple cases. The following may prove as good as anything that we know of for the general run of these cases:

Strychnine Sulphate	12 grains
Fluid Extract of Convallaria	½ ounce
Fluid Extract of Belladonna	½ ounce
Water	2 pints

158 SOME COMMON DISEASES OF THE HORSE

Of this mixture, one ounce should be given three times each day in mild cases, but in severe cases, it may be given every two or three hours. If a complication of the lungs or pneumonia is suspected, the following rubbed into the region over the lungs is of much benefit:

>   Oil of Mustard .... 1 ounce
>   Olive or Cottonseed Oil .... 1 pint

This mixture should be shaken well before using and should not be rubbed too briskly and should not be covered; should not be used oftener than twice daily. The secretions about the eyes and nostrils should be cleaned off with warm water a couple of times each day. In cold weather the animal should be well blanketed and the legs should be properly bandaged.

Bacterins and vaccines will give results in treatment or prevention of this disease; they are very satisfactory when they are properly used; they are worthy of a trial whenever needed. The results will be worth much more than the cost.

When this disease manifests itself in the stable, the sick animals and the well ones should be separated at once and the infected stalls thoroughly cleaned and disinfected. The entire stable should be cleaned and disinfected and there should be a separate attendant for the sick animals. No utensils, clothing, harness, etc., that are used around the sick animals should be used with the well ones. They should be watered separately. Good ventilation and cleanliness will do much to prevent this condition. In all cases of this kind it is always advisable to secure a veterinarian when one can be had.

Strangles or Distemper

This is an acute contagious infectious disease of horses. It is characterized by inflammatory conditions of the respiratory system and also by abscess formation of the superficial lymph glands of the throat.

This disease is found practically at all seasons of the year in the large horse markets. In the rural districts it usually attacks young horses and colts; it may attack horses that are slightly older if they have not already had an attack of the disease. While the percentage of the loss is not high, yet losses do occur and it greatly retards the development of young animals.

This is produced by one of the pus producing germs called the Streptococcus Equi of Schutz.

The infection is carried from animal to animal in the form of the secretions from the affected animals and it gains access to the mucous membranes of the healthy animal by means of the food and water. This secretion adheres to the mucous membranes where it sets up an inflammation. Through the skin it gains access to the blood stream and localizes in the lymph glands of the throat and neck. This disease is carried from one stable to another by horses that have not

160   SOME COMMON DISEASES OF THE HORSE

entirely recovered or animals that are in the earlier stages. It is spread from the market centers through the sale of young animals. A poorly ventilated barn is a predisposing factor to this condition, as the air is moist and not replaced fast enough to prevent the animals rebreathing the air from affected horses; in this way it is much more likely to be carried.

Any object that will carry the discharge is quite apt to be a carrier of this disease—water, feed such as hay, straw and the like, buckets, halters, and any other object that the diseased horse may come in contact with. The attendant is a frequent carrier. Drying lowers the virulence of the secretion, but does not entirely kill it. It is a well known fact that it is a common occurrence in many large stables at about the same time each year. It is almost impossible to disinfect the ordinary barn, so that the infection will be entirely destroyed. With the modern methods of furnishing stables with steel and concrete furnishings, this no doubt can be accomplished.

It is possible that an animal may become infected with this condition by way of the intestinal tract. We do know that the stallion may transmit this condition to the mare during copulation; the suckling colt may also carry the infection to the mare by way of the udder.

The animals that are most often attacked are those that are from one-half to five years old; while animals younger and older than this may become infected, it is not so common. One attack of this disease renders the animal immune to further attacks for several years; it is not likely that many animals have more than one attack.

All those conditions that lessen the vitality and natural resistance to disease are predisposing conditions, such as cold, poorly ventilated stables, sudden changes in temperature, fatigue, during transportation, thin and poorly nourished animals.

If the horse has a cold or is greatly exhausted, it may develop symptoms of the disease after the infection gains access to the body in one to two days; ordinarily the symptoms do not become noticeable until from the fourth to the eighth day. The first symptoms noticed are a diminished appetite, listlessness and an increase in body temperature. Very soon in the attack, symptoms of a nasal catarrh are noticed, such as a highly reddened condition of the membranes lining the nostrils, with a secretion of a clear fluid, which rapidly becomes thick and sticky. There is a pronounced cough and the animal dispels great quantities of the discharge during coughing; the discharge is not so sticky in young colts as it is in older horses. There is usually a sore throat present in this condition.

At about the time the discharge from the nostrils makes its first appearance, a swelling of the lymph glands under the jaw is noticed. This swelling at first is hard and indurated, but hot and painful to the touch. It gradually increases in size and the swelling often gets so great as to interfere with the

162 SOME COMMON DISEASES OF THE HORSE

breathing and eating of the animal. This swelling usually becomes so great that the head is held stiffly and extended. When the swelling reaches a certain size, it may remain stationary for several days, but gradually a softening can be determined. These soft spots may occur in one or in several places while the remainder of the swelling remains hard and firm. If these places are not opened with a sharp knife or lancet, they open of their own accord in a few days; they should be opened as soon as the presence of pus can be detected and a soft place can be determined. After the pus has left this abscess cavity, the swelling rapidly subsides.

The breathing is affected in proportion to the extent that the mucous membranes in the throat are involved. Usually there is a cough present, which in some cases may last a couple of weeks after the abscess breaks.

The heart beat is much faster during the time the abscess is forming. The temperature gets very high, from 104° to 106° F. and remains quite high until the pus has all formed; after this the temperature rapidly returns to normal.

The appetite is very poor, due to the inability to chew and swallow without suffering much pain and also due to the high temperature. The animal is at first constipated but frequently this is changed to a foul smelling diarrhea. The urine is very scanty and very highly colored.

The complications in this condition are very seri-

CONTAGIOUS DISEASES 163

ous. The abscessed lymph glands in the region of the throat are apt to break within the throat and produce inhalation pneumonia by the pus being breathed into the lungs. In some few cases there occurs a swelling and an inflammation of the joints. In other cases, large abscesses may develop internally in the small glands, which may produce a blood poisoning upon rupturing; these abscesses may occur in the brain, lungs, kidneys or any of the internal organs. In some rare cases the lymph glands along the neck may abscess and produce enough pressure on the wind pipe to choke the animal to death; the same results may be found in a few cases when the swelling is very pronounced around the throat.

When the infection remains around the upper air passages and the localization of the abscess is confined chiefly to those glands around the throat, and when the temperature has been high and the abscess formation has been regular the prospects of recovery are very good. The disease usually lasts from two to four weeks; if other parts of the body become affected with abscess formation, it may be longer than this. All those cases in which the abscesses form in other parts of the body, other than around the throat, should be looked upon with suspicion, as they often prove fatal. The general condition and age of the animal has a marked influence, as well as the severity or virulence of the infection. Due to this infection in the region of the throat, many horses are roarers after recovering from strangles.

164 SOME COMMON DISEASES OF THE HORSE

Strangles can be differentiated from other similar conditions by the swelling of the lymph glands under the throat, and from the fact that other horses in the same stable become affected and also from the fact that the disease is present in the community. As soon as the animal is found to be ailing, it should be removed from the well ones; it should be placed in a light, airy, comfortable and well ventilated stall; a box stall if it is available, and it should be well bedded down; comfort should be the first thing in caring for the sick horse. The feed should be easily masticated and, if possible, green, as the animal usually experiences much difficulty owing to the soreness of the throat. Clean fresh water should be kept before the animals all the while. Cleanliness should be the most important consideration in the animal's care; the bedding should be removed daily; the secretion from the eyes and nose should be removed with a soft sponge and warm water at least once or twice each day. The stall should be sprayed with a good disinfectant solution at regular intervals.

It is not often that the disease can be prevented after it has once secured a hold on the animal's body. The most success is to be obtained by hastening the formation of the abscess and liberating the contents as soon as possible. We have always secured the best results with a liniment prepared as follows:

Stronger ammonia water .... 2 ounces
Spirits of Turpentine .... 2 ounces

CONTAGIOUS DISEASES

Oleic Acid .... ½ ounce
Water enough to make 1 quart

This is to be shaken thoroughly and rubbed in well over the surface of the swelling two or three times each day until the abscess is ready to be opened. The abscess should always be opened as soon as possible and always by a veterinarian if one is to be had; if not, an incision fully an inch or an inch and one-half in length should be made just through the skin with a sharp knife that has previously been sterilized by boiling; the index finger is then inserted into this incision and by a series of boring motions, the abscess cavity is punctured and the pus is liberated. The temperature rapidly falls to normal and the swelling rapidly subsides. Great improvement is noticed during the first few hours after the opening of the abscess. For the inflammation of the mouth and the throat, the following will answer very well:

Tincture of iron chloride ...... 1 ounce
Glycerine .... 8 ounces

Place one ounce on the tongue three or four times each day; can be placed on the tongue with a large spoon or dose syringe.

Animals that have had an unusually severe attack and are slow recovering, that have a cough and an irregular appetite, will be greatly benefited by the following:

166 SOME COMMON DISEASES OF THE HORSE

>
> Strychnine sulphate ....12 grains
> Fluid Extract of Belladonna .....½ ounce
> Fluid Extract of Convallria ......½ ounce
> Water .... 1 quart

One ounce three or four times each day with a dose syringe.

Cases that are suffering from extremely difficult breathing can be relieved by the veterinarian who can place a tube in their wind pipe until all danger is past.

This condition should be prevented by the keeping of all young colts and horses away from those animals that are affected and away from all public markets and animals in transit that may carry the disease. In transportation animals should be protected from draughts and storms that may induce colds and thus lower their resistance. Proper ventilation and thorough disinfection will do much to prevent it and also to prevent its recurrence in stables already infected.

Vaccines should be used for prevention of this serious disease of young horses; the early use of vaccines often prevents a severe and costly epidemic.

CHAPTER XVII

MISCELLANEOUS DISEASES

Azoturia or Crick in the Back

By the veterinarian this condition is spoken of as Azoturia, while in many sections the laity speak of it as "Crick in the Back." There is not another disease that has so many terrors for the horse owner and the veterinarian as Azoturia. Veterinarians are agreed as to the diagnosis and usual characteristic symptoms of this condition, but the difference in opinions as to the cause of this condition is as varied as is the treatment of it.

There are several features that stand out prominently in clinical cases of this disease that make it quite difficult to get at the real cause of the trouble. Most of the veterinarians have until the last few years held to the toxemia theory. They thought that it was caused by the absorption or taking up of great quantities of poisonous material into the blood stream, when the excretory organs such as the bowels and kidneys were not working properly. This theory will not stand investigation for any poison that is severe enough to render a horse so completely helpless in such a short time, could not be relieved as quickly as this condition sometimes is, nor would it do so without treatment. Yet we see many mild cases of this condition that would recover in a few hours with no treatment other than absolute rest. This is a cold weather disease as we see much of it during the cooler months of the year, but very little of it during the hot months. It usually occurs after a short period of idleness, and in young growing horses; it does occur, however, in older horses but not with the frequency that it does in younger ones. It is much more severe in city horses than it is in country horses, which is due to the more concentrated feed that they consume and the more violent exercises that they receive. In city horses it often comes on so suddenly that the driver has no warning, before the animal goes down. In country horses, there is usually ample warning that it is coming on, as the symptoms appear before the disease is well established. A larger number of city horses die in proportion to those affected than do country horses.

It remained for a western veterinarian to announce a theory that seems to be the best one that has been offered to date, and one which will stand investigation pretty thoroughly. This has been termed the mechanical theory.

The horse at rest is often fed rich nitrogenous feed that makes the blood thick and heavy. The circulation becomes sluggish, due to the lack of exercise, the great quantity of nitrogenous material in the blood makes the muscles of the blood vessel

MISCELLANEOUS DISEASES

walls flaccid and weak; they do not have their normal elasticity, while on the other hand the nervous system is stimulated and the animal is feeling exceptionally lively. It is a rare thing to see a horse develop Azoturia that has not shown indications just

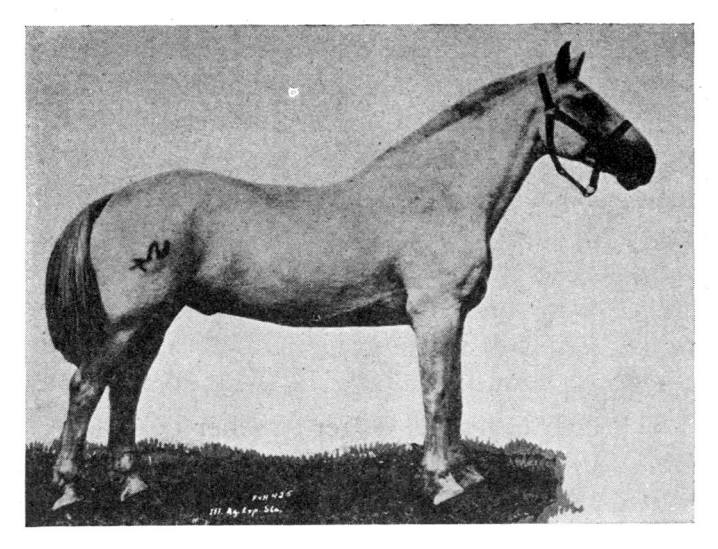

This is how the wormy horse looked a few weeks after being properly treated for the removal of the worms. *Photo Illinois Agricultural Experiment Station.*

previous to taking the attack that he was feeling much better than usual. The horse is taken out to work or for use of any kind, and since he is feeling so good and his nerves are stimulated so highly, and the blood vessels are weaker than they should be, the exercise that he receives for the first few minutes causes his heart to work much faster than usual, pumping large quantities of blood into the blood vessels that are not in any condition to accommodate this extra amount. This condition renders the animal very excitable and produces a paralysis of those particular muscles in which the blood has stopped. In most cases, if the animal is stopped when these symptoms are first noticed, a rapid recovery takes place, as the blood vessels rid themselves of this extra accumulation of blood and the animal returns to normal in a few hours. However, if rest is not given at once, the blood vessels soon become unable to remove the large quantities of blood that are pumped into these parts and it is only a matter of several hours until it has coagulated, and then the animal dies with symptoms similar to apoplexy.

Azoturia manifests itself in a number of ways. Some horses will act very much like a horse with an attack of indigestion, look around toward the flank at frequent intervals and show evidence of quite a little pain, and may even get up and down a few times. Others may show an affection of the muscles of the forelimb or of some other group of muscles. Most of them show a marked lameness in one hind leg, in rare cases in both, and a hard swollen condition of the muscles over the loin. This lameness may be slight at first, but rapidly gets worse. The animal can scarcely walk. The breathing is labored and fast and the animal breaks out into a profuse sweat. If the animal is kept moving, it rapidly

MISCELLANEOUS DISEASES

grows worse and soon goes down unable to rise again. Some animals are so nervous that it is almost impossible to give them medicine by the way of the mouth. City horses usually go down in spite of all the veterinarian may do, but those cases in the country are more mild and many of them, if they receive good care and the proper attention will remain upon their feet throughout the attack. The animal that does not recover sufficiently to get upon its feet in forty-eight hours will very often die. A few will remain down for several days and then recover but these are the exception to the rule.

Horses that go down with this condition should not be put in slings, neither should they be raised up with them, as it generally does more harm than good. Horses that are down should be bedded down well and made as comfortable as possible. They should be turned over every three or four hours. Horses that cannot get upon their feet with the help of a couple of strong men lifting upon the tail, very rarely get up or stay up very long when slings are used. When the attack is coming on, do not fight the horse in an effort to keep it upon its feet. The effort you compel it to put forth in trying to remain upon its feet will only aggravate the condition. If the animal wants to lie down, permit it to do so, and then make it as comfortable as possible. Rest is the most essential thing in the treatment, so stop the animal as soon as the first symptoms are noticed, and keep the animal as quiet as possible. Do not try to make a barn or the village before stopping the animal, but stop wherever you may happen to be. Blanket the animal if the weather makes it necessary and keep it quiet.

Horses that are lightly exercised and then rested for a half hour or so before going to work do not get Azoturia. This light exercise stimulates the circulation and thus prevents any clogging of the blood vessels. Horses in which the grain ration is greatly reduced during idleness and whose bowels and kidneys are kept active by proper feeding very seldom contract this condition. Animals that have been idle for some little time are not as liable to develop Azoturia as those that have been idle but a day or so. Horses idle for several days have this disease in a milder form. Mares do not have this disease as severely as geldings do, and the percentage of recoveries is much higher among them.

It has been the common belief among most people that the urine of all horses affected with Azoturia is always dark colored, but such is not the case. For the first several hours of the attack, the urine may be almost normal in color, but if recovery does not begin within a few hours, the urine turns dark, sometimes being almost as dark in color as coffee. Many people are of the opinion that it is always necessary to draw the urine, but we seldom follow that procedure any more and we feel that our results are better than they were when we followed the prac-

MISCELLANEOUS DISEASES

tice of drawing the urine early in the attack. It has been our experience that if you get the animal into a comfortable position and resting as it should, it will only be an hour or so until it will void the urine of its own volition.

When an animal is known to be susceptible to this condition, or when it shows by its actions that something is wrong, especially if it has been idle for a day or so, it is well to suspect Azoturia. The animal should be stopped at once and kept just as quiet as possible. Send for a veterinarian at once, for some cases that appear very mild and seem to be getting along very well very suddenly take a relapse and go down. Do not take any chances, as they are frequently the cause of the loss of a valuable animal.

If you have an animal that is subject to these attacks, cut down the grain ration at least one-half, when the animal is to be idle for a day or so, and see to it that the animal has some exercise each day. If, for any reason, it is not possible to exercise for a day or so, exercise for a few minutes and then allow the animal to rest a half hour before putting to work. Keep the bowels free by the use of oil meal or bran.

There is no treatment that is a specific, and the proper care and attention that should be given by the owner early in the attack and the care during the attack will many times contribute more to the recovery than anything else that can be done.

Tetanus or Lock Jaw

This condition, as it is commonly found, is quite pronounced and when once seen it is easily recognized whenever and wherever it may be seen. It is so called from the fact that the muscles become very

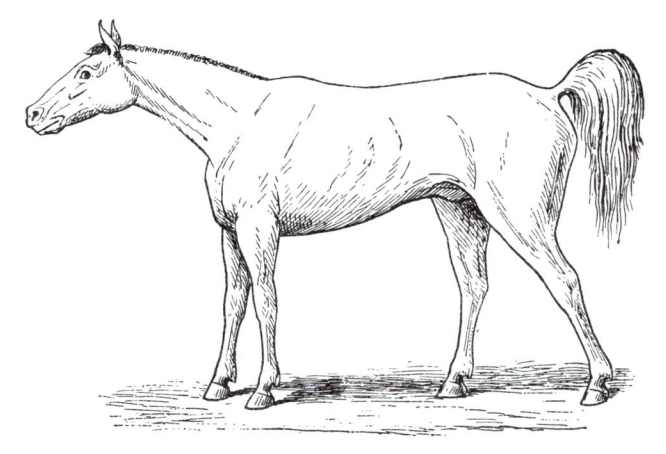

This is a typical appearance of a horse with lock jaw (tetanus).

rigid and undergo violent contraction, to the extent that the animal's jaws frequently become locked, preventing the animal's eating and drinking.

This condition is caused by a germ that usually finds its way into a deep seated wound from a small slender object. It rarely happens in large open well-drained wounds, since it will not grow in the presence of air. For this reason, nail wounds, pitchfork

MISCELLANEOUS DISEASES

wounds, and the like usually are the cause of such a condition. Every wound that is deep and in which a good circulation of air is impossible should be opened thoroughly to provide drainage and then the animal should be treated to prevent this disease.

The animal with tetanus will first be noticed having difficulty of eating, have a stilty gait, slobber slightly and is usually nervous. If the head is raised slightly, a membrane covers a part of the eye ball and this is a never failing symptom. The animal has difficulty lifting its feet off the ground. Breathing is fast and shallow and drinking and eating rapidly become more difficult.

Whenever a horse has an injury of the nature given above, it should have a prophylactic dose of tetanus antitoxin. If this is given in the proper sized dose within a few hours after the injury, it is practically 100 per cent effective.

This condition may develop in two to five days after the injury but usually it is a week or even ten days. The quicker it develops, the less chance the animal has, for this indicates that the germ is very virulent. A good veterinarian should be called early, but if the proper dose of tetanus antitoxin had been given, this would not be necessary.

CHAPTER XVIII

DISEASES OF YOUNG FOALS

In many sections of the country the breeders of horses have had much difficulty in the successful rearing of their foals. As long as draft horses remain as high in price as they are at this time, the loss of a foal from a well-bred draft stallion and a good dam would represent the loss of about fifty dollars at least and in some cases much more than this. Much of these losses can be prevented if the proper methods are observed by the owner or caretaker at the time of the colt's birth, and also a few days before and after the same.

The one disease among foals that causes great losses is known as Navel Ill, or Joint Disease. This is an infectious disease and by observing proper and thorough sanitary precautions this loss could be very greatly reduced. Another condition that causes great loss is acute intestinal catarrh or diarrhea.

Caring for the Mare

The mare that is about to foal should receive special care and should not be treated as though she would not foal. For the last two or three weeks the mare should be fed so that the bowels are loose and

DISEASES OF YOUNG FOALS

should be fed only easily digestible feed and not in too large quantities. She should have exercise in the open when possible every day. Light work will do no harm, but if it is not absolutely necessary the mare

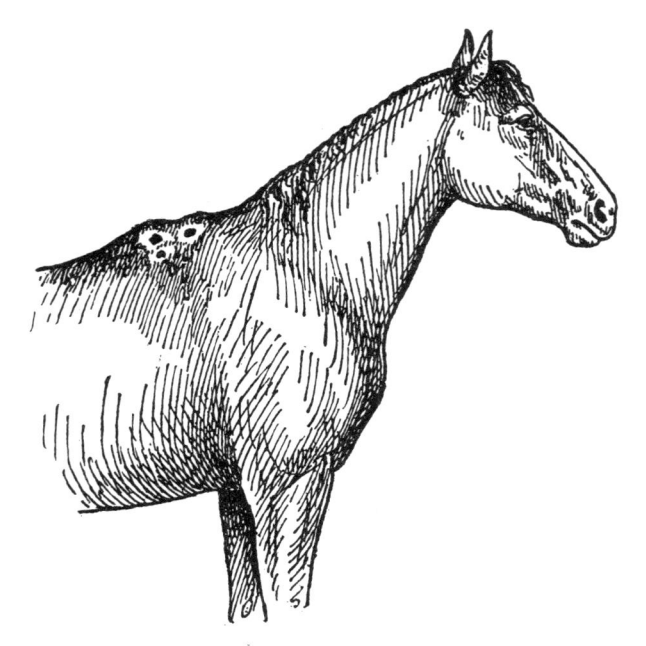

This shows the location of fistula of the withers.

would do better and the risk would be greatly lessened if she was not worked at all during the last two or three weeks. If a mare should be worked hard right up to the time of foaling and has a normal foal without any complication it would possibly do her no harm, and we have known of several of them that were worked up to foaling time, but if she should happen to have a difficult foaling time and require some assistance, she will be very liable to complications and she will not come through the ordeal as good as she might have done had she had her natural strength, instead of being worked down.

It is good business to have someone about when the mare foals, as often the afterbirth is so dense that the foal is unable to rupture it by its weight when it falls, or when the mother gets on her feet and many a colt smothers because there is no one present to rupture the membranes.

The last two or three weeks of the mare's time she should be placed in a clean box stall and it should be thoroughly cleaned and disinfected and should be kept well bedded with clean straw. Other animals, and especially any that have bad suppurating wounds or sores should not be permitted in this part of the barn. It is well to have a stall in the barn for this purpose and then keep it in good shape.

Diarrhea or Acute Intestinal Catarrh

The stomach and the bowels of the young foals are very delicate and sensitive and are very susceptible to digestive disturbances. An improper composition of the milk due to improper feeding of the mother sometimes is very detrimental to the foal and causes this digestive disturbance. Feeding the mother feed that is green or that is particularly rich or feed that is

DISEASES OF YOUNG FOALS

succulent and watery, or feed that is spoiled or that is laxative will often times have a bad effect on the foal. There are a few diseases of the mother that may affect the foal through the milk, such as indigestion, inflammation of the udder or any of the contagious or infectious diseases. Overexertion of the mother sometimes disturbs the secretion of the milk so that this condition is brought about. The foal should not be kept from the mare too long at a time as it is then apt to overload the stomach. The young should be kept in a warm, comfortable place and should not be kept in a cold damp stable. The foal should always be allowed to nurse the first milk when at all possible as this acts as a laxative for it.

The first thing that is usually noticed is that the foal does not care to nurse and if put to the mare it will nurse a little or maybe none at all, and will then seem dull and drowsy and maybe a little fever will be present. Soon a diarrhea is noticed. Sometimes this gradually gets worse until this diarrhea becomes a thin watery fluid and the foal will strain when it is voided. This is yellowish and later becomes grayish in color and is frequently streaked with blood. It has a disagreeable sour smell. If diarrhea persists the foal becomes very weak and loses flesh rapidly.

The majority of these cases recover. But occasionally one will die in two or three days and sometimes one will linger for several weeks and then finally die.

The first thing and the most important is the regulation of the diet of the mother and the proper care of her. See, first, that the mare is receiving the proper care. See that other conditions, such as stabling and the like, are favorable. If the condition is not grave at the beginning, and can be readily traced to errors in dieting or caring for the mother, get equal parts of zinc and sodium sulphorcarbolates and give the foal, dissolved in a little water, three or four times each day, one-half teaspoonful of this mixture. Or ten or fifteen drops of formalin dissolved in a pint of sweet milk and given to the foal two or three times each day. This is commonly spoken of as formaldehyde.

Navel Ill or Joint Evil

This is a contagious disease of foals that annually causes great losses to the breeder. It usually shows up within the first couple of days after the colt is born and never later than the fourth week after birth. It is usually characterized by a swelling of the joints which are filled with pus.

This disease is found in some sections and occurs from year to year. It is caused by a germ that is easily carried by other animals and in the buildings and occasionally in the mother's own body. This condition usually is contracted after the foal is born but it may be possible for the foal to take the disease from the mother while she has been affected with some contagious disease, such as influenza or from infection that gains access during birth. The infection gains access through the navel stump.

The navel stump of the new-born is wet and covered with blood and is filled with a jelly-like substance and as the circulation is cut off it makes a fertile place for the development of any bacteria that may come into contact with it. Foals that are

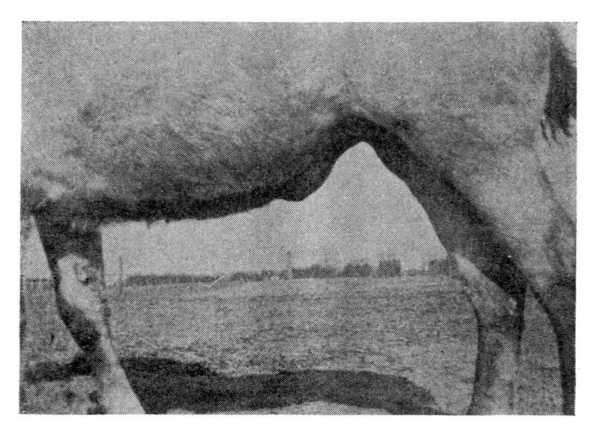

Navel rupture is quite common in young foals. Should be repaired by a competent veterinarian when colt is but a few weeks of age. *Courtesy Prof. R. S. Hudson, Michigan State College.*

affected will soil the straw and bedding and foals that are then born and come in contact with this soiled bedding are apt to contract the disease through the improperly cared for navel stump.

The navel is moist and does not dry up as rapidly as usual. A small swelling appears at the navel and this appears hot to the touch. The colt does not move about a great deal and when it does it is with

182 SOME COMMON DISEASES OF THE HORSE

difficulty and very slowly. It does not have the normal desire for nursing and a slight temperature develops. If treated early some cases will improve rapidly while other symptoms will gradually become more severe and those of a general blood poisoning occur. Usually at this time some of the joints become swollen and the animal goes lame. It is usually the hock or knee joint that is first affected. If this infection can not be checked the joint will eventually break and will discharge a sticky pus. This condition is usually subject to complications and sometimes a pneumonia develops which is ushered in by difficult breathing and a hard dry cough and a discharge from the nose. Death usually follows this complication in a very short time. Digestive disturbances are almost always present with this condition.

Some of these cases die in two or three days, while some of the others will linger along into the chronic stage. The average will possibly linger from two to three weeks. The mortality is very high, running on an average of about one-half.

The treatment of this condition must only be attempted by a competent veterinarian, but many times this can be prevented by caring for the mare and fixing quarters such as was recommended in the fore part of this article and the proper care of the animal as soon as it is born. The navel cord should not be ligated or tied, but it should be rendered as near antiseptic as possible and dried up as rapidly as possible. If the stump of the cord is painted every fifteen minutes with formalin for three or four hours it will usually be pretty well dried up by the end of that time. There is very little danger after the cord is once dry. It may also be painted three or four times for the first day or so with iodine collodion or it may be painted the same number of times daily with tincture of iodine. The proper and prompt care of the navel stump will prevent the larger number of these conditions. This disinfection of the stump of the navel cord should be done thoroughly and carefully and if you have had the disease on the place in the neighborhood and have never taken care of such a case it would be well to call on your veterinarian and have him give you specific directions as to just how to care for the colt when he is born. It may save you a valuable foal.

Not all the losses in foals are caused from these two conditions but the larger part of them are, and we feel quite sure that if you make a conscientious effort to prevent these two conditions that you will have removed the greater part of your danger of losing your spring foals. Try it.

INDEX

Azoturia (crick in the back), 167

Bedding the Horse, 40
Bedding, the Purpose of, 42
Bedding, Straw as a, 42
Bedding, the Use of Sawdust as, 45
Blanket, the Type of, 37
Blanket, the Fit of the, 39
Blanket, the Use and Abuse of the, 40
Breathing (Respiratory) Diseases, 127
  Cold in Head, 127
  Treatment of Cold in Head, 128
  Bronchitis, 129
  Treatment of Bronchitis, 130
  Congestion of Lungs, 130
  Pneumonia (Lung Fever), 131
  Heaves, 133
Bronchitis, 129

Capped Elbow, 137
Care of the Sick Horse, 110
  Make the Horse Comfortable, 111
  Clothing (Blanketing), 113
  Feeding and Watering, 114
Causes of Disease, 56
  Inherited, 87
  Exciting, 88
  Specific, 90
Clipping the Horse, 79
  Winter Coat, the, 79
  Purpose of, 81
  The Clipping Operation, 82
  The Time for, 84
  Winter, the Effect of, 85
Colic (Indigestion), 117
  Acute, 118

Treatment of Acute, 122
Impaction, 122
Treatment of Impaction, 124
Contagious Diseases, 151
  Influenza, 151
  Treatment of Influenza, 157
  Strangles (Distemper), 159
  Treatment of Strangles, 164
Cold in the Head, 127
Congestion of Lungs, 130
Corns, 140
Crowding in Stall, 53
Curb, 144
Curry Combs and Their Use, 59

Danby Brush, 61
Diarrhea (Scours), 125
  Treatment of, 126
Doors of Stable, 25
Dose Syringe, 106
Drainage of Stable, 26
Drenching, 104
Drinking Water, Medicine in, 108

Eating Manure, 55

Feeding, Effect of in Condition, 100
Feed Carrier, 28
Feet, Care of, 144
Feet and Legs, 135
  Sweeney of Shoulder, 137
  Capped Elbow, 137
  Splint, 138
  Ringbones, 138
  Sidebones, 139
  Sand Cracks (Hoof Cracks), 140
  Corns, 140
  Foundered Hoof, 141

INDEX

Thrush, 141
Thoroughpin, 142
Bog Spavin, 142
Bone Spavin, 143
Curb, 144
Care of Feet, 144
Floor of Stable, 21
Foals, Diseases of Young, 176
Foundered Hoof, 141

Gnawing the Walls, 55
Grooming, 57
  Tools for, 59
  Curry Combs and Their Use, 59
  Water Brush, 61
  Dandy Brush, 55
  Sponges, 62
  Rubbing Cloths, 62
  Sweat Scraper, 62
  Mane Combs, 63
  Time for, 63
  Methods of, 64
  Brushing the Mane, 65
  Thinning the Mane, 68
  Laying the Mane, 68

Halter, the Fitting of, 30
Halter, Slipping the, 34
Heaves, 133
How to Handle the Horse, 69
  Twitch, the Use of, 70
  War and Pulley Bridle, 72
  Taking up the Foreleg, 75
  Squeeze or Crowding, 75
  Side Line, 77

Impaction, 122
Influenza of the Horse, 151

Kicking in the Stable, 52

Latches, Catches, Etc., for Barn, 25
Litter Carrier, 27
Location of Stable, 15
Lung Fever (Pneumonia), 131

Mane, the Laying of the, 68
Mane, Thinning, 68

Mane, Brushing the, 65
Mane Combs, 63
Manger, 24
Manger, Fastening Horse to the, 32
Medicines, How to Give, 103
  Drenching, 104
  Dose Syringe, 106
  Use of Capsule, 107
  With the Grain, 108
  In the Drinking Water, 108
  On the Tongue, 109

Navel Ill of Foals, 180

Pneumonia (Lung Fever), 131
Prevention of Disease, 96
  Condition in, 98
  Amount and Kind of Work, 99
  Effect of Feeding in, 100
  Features of Early Training in, 101
Pulse Rate of Horse, 95

Ringbones, 138

Sand Cracks, 140
Scours (Diarrhea), 125
  Treatment of, 126
Sick Horse—How to Tell, 92
Sidebones, 139
Spavin-Bone, 143
Spavin-Bog, 142
Splint, 138
Stable and Its Equipment, 15
  Location of, 15
  Ventilation of, 17
  Materials Used for, 20
  Floor of, 21
  Windows of, 22
  Stalls of, 23
  Manger of, 24
  Hay Racks of, 24
  Doors of, 25
  Latches, Catches, Etc., 25
  Drainage of, 26
  Litter Carrier, 27
  Feed Carrier, 28
Strangles, 159

INDEX

Sweeney of the Shoulder, 137

Tearing the Clothing, 54
Temperature of Horse, 95
Tetanus (Lock-Jaw), 174
Thrush, 141
Tricks and Vices of the Horse, 47
  Weaving, 49
  Windsucking, 50
  Crib-Biting, 50
  Kicking, 52

Crowding in Stall, 53
Biting, 54
Tearing the Clothing, 54
Gnawing the Walls, 55
Eating Manure, 55
Twitch, the Use of, 70
Tying—Cross in Stable, 36

War & Pulley Bridle, 72
Weaving, 49
Windsucking, 50

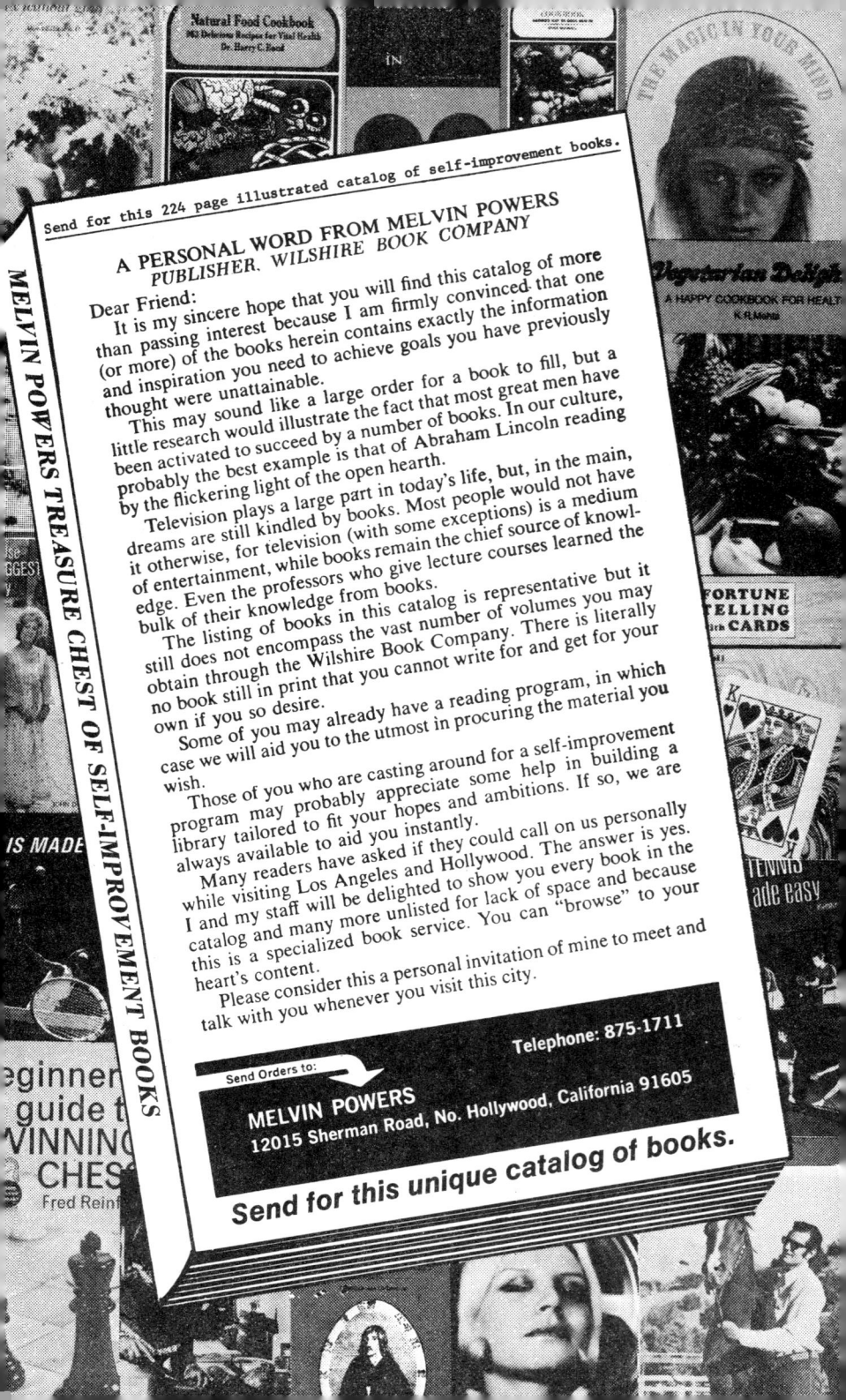

Send for this 224 page illustrated catalog of self-improvement books.

A PERSONAL WORD FROM MELVIN POWERS
PUBLISHER, WILSHIRE BOOK COMPANY

Dear Friend:

It is my sincere hope that you will find this catalog of more than passing interest because I am firmly convinced that one (or more) of the books herein contains exactly the information and inspiration you need to achieve goals you have previously thought were unattainable.

This may sound like a large order for a book to fill, but a little research would illustrate the fact that most great men have been activated to succeed by a number of books. In our culture, probably the best example is that of Abraham Lincoln reading by the flickering light of the open hearth.

Television plays a large part in today's life, but, in the main, dreams are still kindled by books. Most people would not have it otherwise, for television (with some exceptions) is a medium of entertainment, while books remain the chief source of knowledge. Even the professors who give lecture courses learned the bulk of their knowledge from books.

The listing of books in this catalog is representative but it still does not encompass the vast number of volumes you may obtain through the Wilshire Book Company. There is literally no book still in print that you cannot write for and get for your own if you so desire.

Some of you may already have a reading program, in which case we will aid you to the utmost in procuring the material you wish.

Those of you who are casting around for a self-improvement program may probably appreciate some help in building a library tailored to fit your hopes and ambitions. If so, we are always available to aid you instantly.

Many readers have asked if they could call on us personally while visiting Los Angeles and Hollywood. The answer is yes. I and my staff will be delighted to show you every book in the catalog and many more unlisted for lack of space and because this is a specialized book service. You can "browse" to your heart's content.

Please consider this a personal invitation of mine to meet and talk with you whenever you visit this city.

Telephone: 875-1711

Send Orders to:
MELVIN POWERS
12315 Sherman Road, No. Hollywood, California 91605

Send for this unique catalog of books.

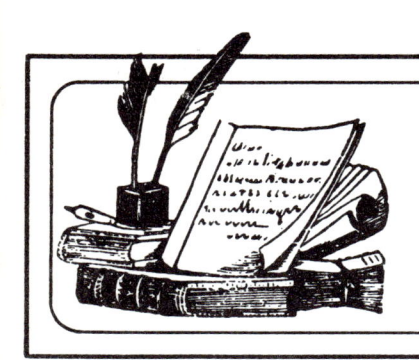

Melvin Powers SELF-IMPROVEMENT LIBRARY

MELVIN POWERS SELF-IMPROVEMENT LIBRARY

____ABILITY TO LOVE Dr. Allan Fromme	$2.00
____ACT YOUR WAY TO SUCCESSFUL LIVING Neil & Margaret Rau	2.00
____ADVANCED TECHNIQUES OF HYPNOSIS Melvin Powers	1.00
____ANIMAL HYPNOSIS Dr. F. A. Völgyesi	2.00
____ARCHERY — An Expert's Guide Don Stamp	2.00
____ASTROLOGY: A FASCINATING HISTORY P. Naylor	2.00
____ASTROLOGY: HOW TO CHART YOUR HOROSCOPE Max Heindel	2.00
____ASTROLOGY: YOUR PERSONAL SUN-SIGN GUIDE Beatrice Ryder	2.00
____ASTROLOGY FOR EVERYDAY LIVING Janet Harris	2.00
____ASTROLOGY GUIDE TO GOOD HEALTH Alexandra Kayhle	2.00
____ASTROLOGY MADE EASY Astarte	2.00
____ASTROLOGY MADE PRACTICAL Alexandra Kayhle	2.00
____ASTROLOGY, ROMANCE, YOU AND THE STARS Anthony Norvell	2.00
____BEGINNER'S GUIDE TO WINNING CHESS Fred Reinfeld	2.00
____BETTER CHESS — How to Play Fred Reinfeld	2.00
____BICYCLING FOR FUN AND GOOD HEALTH Kenneth E. Luther	2.00
____BOOK OF TALISMANS, AMULETS & ZODIACAL GEMS William Pavitt	3.00
____BRIDGE BIDDING MADE EASY Edwin Kantar	5.00
____BRIDGE CONVENTIONS Edwin Kantar	4.00
____CHECKERS MADE EASY Tom Wiswell	2.00
____CHESS IN TEN EASY LESSONS Larry Evans	2.00
____CHESS MADE EASY Milton L. Hanauer	2.00
____CHESS MASTERY — A New Approach Fred Reinfeld	2.00
____CHESS PROBLEMS FOR BEGINNERS edited by Fred Reinfeld	2.00
____CHESS SECRETS REVEALED Fred Reinfeld	2.00
____CHESS STRATEGY — An Expert's Guide Fred Reinfeld	2.00
____CHESS TACTICS FOR BEGINNERS edited by Fred Reinfeld	2.00
____CHESS THEORY & PRACTICE Morry & Mitchell	2.00
____CHILDBIRTH WITH HYPNOSIS William S. Kroger, M.D.	2.00
____COIN COLLECTING FOR BEGINNERS Burton Hobson & Fred Reinfeld	2.00
____COMPLETE GUIDE TO FISHING Vlad Evanoff	2.00
____CONCENTRATION—A Guide to Mental Mastery Mouni Sadhu	2.00
____CONVERSATION MADE EASY Elliot Russell	2.00
____CULPEPER'S HERBAL REMEDIES Dr. Nicholas Culpeper	2.00
____CYBERNETICS WITHIN US Y. Saparina	3.00
____DOCTOR PSYCHO-CYBERNETICS Maxwell Maltz, M.D.	2.50
____DOG TRAINING MADE EASY & FUN John W. Kellogg	2.00
____DREAMS & OMENS REVEALED Fred Gettings	2.00
____DR. LINDNER'S SPECIAL WEIGHT CONTROL METHOD	1.00
____DYNAMIC THINKING Melvin Powers	1.00

ENCYCLOPEDIA OF MODERN SEX & LOVE TECHNIQUES R. Macandrew	2.00
EXAM SECRET Dennis B. Jackson	2.00
EXTRASENSORY PERCEPTION Simeon Edmunds	2.00
FAST GOURMET COOKBOOK Poppy Cannon	2.50
400 FASCINATING MAGIC TRICKS YOU CAN DO Howard Thurston	2.00
FORTUNE TELLING WITH CARDS P. Foli	2.00
GAYELORD HAUSER'S NEW GUIDE TO INTELLIGENT REDUCING	3.00
GOULD'S GOLD & SILVER GUIDE TO COINS Maurice Gould	2.00
GREATEST POWER IN THE UNIVERSE U. S. Andersen	4.00
GROW RICH WHILE YOU SLEEP Ben Sweetland	2.00
GUIDE TO DEVELOPING YOUR POTENTIAL Herbert A. Otto, Ph.D.	3.00
GUIDE TO HAPPINESS Dr. Maxwell S. Cagan	2.00
GUIDE TO LIVING IN BALANCE Frank S. Caprio, M.D.	2.00
GUIDE TO RATIONAL LIVING Albert Ellis, Ph.D. & R. Harper, Ph.D.	2.00
GUIDE TO SUCCESSFUL MARRIAGE Drs. Albert Ellis & Robert Harper	3.00
HANDWRITING ANALYSIS MADE EASY John Marley	2.00
HANDWRITING TELLS Nadya Olyanova	3.00
HARMONICA PLAYING FOR FUN & PROFIT Hal Leighton	2.00
HEALING POWER OF HERBS May Bethel	2.00
HELP YOURSELF TO BETTER SIGHT Margaret Darst Corbett	2.00
HELPING YOURSELF WITH APPLIED PSYCHOLOGY R. Henderson	2.00
HELPING YOURSELF WITH PSYCHIATRY Frank S. Caprio, M.D.	2.00
HERB HANDBOOK Dawn MacLeod	2.00
HERBS FOR COOKING AND HEALING Dr. Donald Law	2.00
HERBS FOR HEALTH How to Grow & Use Them Louise Evans Doole	2.00
HOME GARDEN COOKBOOK Delicious Natural Food Recipes Ken Kraft	3.00
HOW TO ATTRACT GOOD LUCK A. H. Z. Carr	2.00
HOW TO BE A COMEDIAN FOR FUN & PROFIT King & Laufer	2.00
HOW TO CONTROL YOUR DESTINY Norvell	2.00
HOW TO DEVELOP A BETTER SPEAKING VOICE M. Hellier	2.00
HOW TO DEVELOP A WINNING PERSONALITY Martin Panzer	2.00
HOW TO DEVELOP AN EXCEPTIONAL MEMORY Young and Gibson	2.00
HOW TO IMPROVE YOUR BRIDGE Alfred Sheinwold	2.00
HOW TO IMPROVE YOUR VISION Dr. Robert A. Kraskin	2.00
HOW TO LIVE A RICHER & FULLER LIFE Rabbi Edgar F. Magnin	2.00
HOW TO MAKE A FORTUNE IN REAL ESTATE Albert Winnikoff	3.00
HOW TO MAKE MONEY IN REAL ESTATE Stanley L. McMichael	2.00
HOW TO OVERCOME YOUR FEARS M. P. Leahy, M.D.	2.00
HOW TO RAISE AN EMOTIONALLY HEALTHY, HAPPY CHILD Albert Ellis, Ph.D.	2.00
HOW TO SLEEP WITHOUT PILLS Dr. David F. Tracy	1.00
HOW TO SOLVE YOUR SEX PROBLEMS WITH SELF-HYPNOSIS Frank S. Caprio, M.D.	2.00
HOW TO STOP SMOKING THRU SELF-HYPNOSIS Leslie M. LeCron	2.00
HOW TO UNDERSTAND YOUR DREAMS Geoffrey A. Dudley	2.00
HOW TO USE AUTO-SUGGESTION EFFECTIVELY John Duckworth	2.00
HOW TO WIN AT CHECKERS Fred Reinfeld	2.00
HOW TO WIN AT POCKET BILLIARDS Edward D. Knuchell	2.00
HOW TO WIN AT POKER Terence Reese & Anthony T. Watkins	2.00
HOW TO WIN AT THE RACES Sam (The Genius) Lewin	2.00
HOW YOU CAN BOWL BETTER USING SELF-HYPNOSIS Jack Heise	2.00
HOW YOU CAN HAVE CONFIDENCE AND POWER Les Giblin	2.00
HOW YOU CAN PLAY BETTER GOLF USING SELF-HYPNOSIS Heise	2.00
HOW YOU CAN STOP SMOKING PERMANENTLY Ernest Caldwell	2.00
HYPNOSIS AND SELF-HYPNOSIS Bernard Hollander, M.D.	2.00
HYPNOSIS IN ATHLETICS Wilfred M. Mitchell, Ph.D.	2.00
HYPNOTISM (Originally published in 1893) Carl Sextus	3.00

____HYPNOTISM & PSYCHIC PHENOMENA Simeon Edmunds		2.00
____HYPNOTISM MADE EASY Dr. Ralph Winn		2.00
____HYPNOTISM MADE PRACTICAL Louis Orton		2.00
____HYPNOTISM REVEALED Melvin Powers		1.00
____HYPNOTISM TODAY Leslie LeCron & Jean Bordeaux, Ph.D.		2.00
____HYPNOTIST'S CASE BOOK Alex Erskine		1.00
____I WILL Ben Sweetland		2.00
____ILLUSTRATED YOGA William Zorn		2.00
____IMPOTENCE & FRIGIDITY Edwin W. Hirsch, M.D.		2.00
____INCREASE YOUR LEARNING POWER Geoffrey A. Dudley		2.00
____JUGGLING MADE EASY Rudolf Dittrich		1.00
____LEFT-HANDED PEOPLE Michael Barsley		3.00
____LSD – THE AGE OF MIND Bernard Roseman		2.00
____MAGIC IN YOUR MIND U. S. Andersen		2.00
____MAGIC MADE EASY Byron Wels		2.00
____MAGIC OF NUMBERS Robert Tocquet		2.00
____MAGIC OF THINKING BIG Dr. David J. Schwartz		2.00
____MAGIC POWER OF YOUR MIND Walter M. Germain		2.00
____MAGICIAN – His training and work W. E. Butler		2.00
____MASTER KEYS TO SUCCESS, POPULARITY & PRESTIGE C. W. Bailey		2.00
____MEDICAL HYPNOSIS HANDBOOK Drs. Van Pelt, Ambrose, Newbold		2.00
____MEDITATION Mouni Sadhu		3.00
____MENTAL POWER THRU SLEEP SUGGESTION Melvin Powers		1.00
____MENTAL TELEPATHY EXPLAINED Hereward Carrington		.50
____MIND OVER PLATTER Peter G. Lindner, M.D.		2.00
____MODERN HYPNOSIS Lesley Kuhn & Salvatore Russo, Ph.D.		3.00
____MODERN ISRAEL Lily Edelman		2.00
____MODERN NUMEROLOGY Morris C. Goodman		2.00
____MOTORCYCLING FOR BEGINNERS I. G. Edmonds		2.00
____MY WORLD OF ASTROLOGY Sydney Omarr		2.00
____NATURAL FOOD COOKBOOK Dr. Harry C. Bond		2.00
____NATURE'S MEDICINES Richard Lucas		2.00
____NEW APPROACHES TO SEX IN MARRIAGE John E. Eichelaub, M.D.		2.00
____NEW CARBOHYDRATE DIET COUNTER Patti Lopez-Pereira		1.00
____NEW CONCEPTS OF HYPNOSIS Bernard C. Gindes, M.D.		3.00
____NUMEROLOGY—ITS FACTS AND SECRETS Ariel Yvon Taylor		2.00
____1001 BRILLIANT WAYS TO CHECKMATE Fred Reinfeld		2.00
____1001 WINNING CHESS SACRIFICES & COMBINATIONS Fred Reinfeld		2.00
____ORIENTAL SECRETS OF GRACEFUL LIVING Boye De Mente		1.00
____OUR JEWISH HERITAGE Rabbi Alfred Wolf & Joseph Gaer		2.00
____PALMISTRY MADE EASY Fred Gettings		2.00
____PALMISTRY MADE PRACTICAL Elizabeth Daniels Squire		2.00
____PALMISTRY SECRETS REVEALED Henry Frith		2.00
____PEYOTE STORY Bernard Roseman		2.00
____PIGEONS: HOW TO RAISE AND TRAIN THEM William H. Allen, Jr.		2.00
____POST-HYPNOTIC INSTRUCTIONS Arnold Furst		2.00
How to give post-hypnotic suggestions for therapeutic purposes.		
____PRACTICAL BOATING W. S. Kals		3.00
____PRACTICAL GUIDE TO BETTER CONCENTRATION Melvin Powers		2.00
____PRACTICAL GUIDE TO PUBLIC SPEAKING Maurice Forley		2.00
____PRACTICAL GUIDE TO SELF-HYPNOSIS Melvin Powers		2.00
____PRACTICAL HYPNOTISM Philip Magonet, M.D.		1.00
____PRACTICAL YOGA Ernest Wood		2.00
____PROPHECY IN OUR TIME Martin Ebon		2.50
____PSYCH YOURSELF TO BETTER TENNIS Dr. Walter A. Luszki		2.00
____PSYCHEDELIC ECSTASY William Marshall & Gilbert W. Taylor		2.00
____PSYCHO-CYBERNETICS Maxwell Maltz, M.D.		2.00
____PSYCHOLOGY OF HANDWRITING Nadya Olyanova		2.00

PSYCHOSOMATIC GYNECOLOGY *William S. Kroger, M.D.*		10.00
ROMANCE OF HASSIDISM *Jacob S. Minkin*		2.50
SECRET OF BOWLING STRIKES *Dawson Taylor*		2.00
SECRET OF PERFECT PUTTING *Horton Smith & Dawson Taylor*		2.00
SECRET OF SECRETS *U. S. Andersen*		3.00
SECRETS OF HYPNOTISM *S. J. Van Pelt, M.D.*		2.00
SEEING INTO THE FUTURE *Harvey Day*		2.00
SELF-CONFIDENCE THROUGH SELF-ANALYSIS *E. Oakley*		1.00
SELF-HYPNOSIS *Paul Adams*		2.00
SELF-HYPNOSIS Its Theory, Technique & Application *Melvin Powers*		2.00
SELF-HYPNOSIS A Conditioned-Response Technique *Laurance Sparks*		2.00
SERVICE OF THE HEART *Evelyn Garfield, Ph.D.*		2.50
7 DAYS TO FASTER READING *William S. Schaill*		2.00
SEW SIMPLY, SEW RIGHT *Mini Rhea & F. Leighton*		2.00
SEX & HUMAN BEHAVIOR BY THE NUMBERS *Alexandra Kayhle*		2.00
SEX WITHOUT GUILT *Albert Ellis, Ph.D.*		2.00
SEXUALLY ADEQUATE FEMALE *Frank S. Caprio, M.D.*		2.00
SEXUALLY ADEQUATE MALE *Frank S. Caprio, M.D.*		2.00
STAMP COLLECTING FOR BEGINNERS *Burton Hobson*		2.00
STAMP COLLECTING FOR FUN & PROFIT *Frank Cetin*		1.00
STORY OF ISRAEL IN COINS *Jean & Maurice Gould*		2.00
STORY OF ISRAEL IN STAMPS *Maxim & Gabriel Shamir*		1.00
STUDENT'S GUIDE TO BETTER GRADES *J. A. Rickard*		2.00
STUDENT'S GUIDE TO EFFICIENT STUDY *D. E. James*		1.00
STUTTERING AND WHAT YOU CAN DO ABOUT IT *W. Johnson, Ph.D.*		2.00
SUCCESS-CYBERNETICS *U. S. Andersen*		2.00
SUPERSTITION — Are you superstitious? *Eric Maple*		2.00
TABLE TENNIS MADE EASY *Johnny Leach*		2.00
TAROT *Mouni Sadhu*		3.00
TAROT OF THE BOHEMIANS *Papus*		3.00
10 DAYS TO A GREAT NEW LIFE *William E. Edwards*		2.00
TENNIS MADE EASY *Joel Brecheen*		2.00
TEST YOUR ESP *Martin Ebon*		2.00
THERAPY THROUGH HYPNOSIS edited by *Raphael H. Rhodes*		3.00
THINK AND GROW RICH *Napoleon Hill*		2.00
THOUGHT DIAL *Sydney Omarr*		2.00
THREE MAGIC WORDS *U. S. Andersen*		3.00
TONGUE OF THE PROPHETS *Robert St. John*		3.00
TREASURY OF COMFORT edited by *Rabbi Sidney Greenberg*		2.00
TREASURY OF THE ART OF LIVING edited by *Rabbi S. Greenberg*		2.00
VEGETABLE GARDENING FOR BEGINNERS *Hugh Wiberg*		2.00
VEGETABLES FOR TODAY'S GARDENS *R. Milton Carleton*		2.00
VEGETARIAN COOKERY *Janet Walker*		2.00
VEGETARIAN COOKING MADE EASY & DELECTABLE *Veronica Vezza*		2.00
VEGETARIAN DELIGHTS — A Happy Cookbook for Health *K. R. Mehta*		2.00
VEGETARIAN GOURMET COOKBOOK *Joyce McKinnel*		2.00
WAYS TO SELF-REALIZATION *Mounhi Sadhu*		2.00
WITCHCRAFT, MAGIC & OCCULTISM—A Fascinating History *W. B. Crow*		3.00
WITCHCRAFT—THE SIX SENSE *Justine Glass*		2.00
WORLD OF PSYCHIC RESEARCH *Hereward Carrington*		2.00
YOU ARE NOT THE TARGET *Laura Huxley*		3.00
YOU CAN ANALYZE HANDWRITING *Robert Holder*		2.00
YOU CAN LEARN TO RELAX *Dr. Samuel Gutwirth*		2.00
YOUR FIRST YEAR OF MARRIAGE *Dr. Tom McGinnis*		2.00
YOUR SUBCONSCIOUS POWER *Charles M. Simmons*		2.00
YOUR THOUGHTS CAN CHANGE YOUR LIFE *Donald Curtis*		2.00
YOUR WILL & WHAT TO DO ABOUT IT *Attorney Samuel G. Kling*		2.00
ZODIAC REVEALED *Rupert Gleadow*		2.00

PSYCHO-CYBERNETICS
A New Technique for Using Your Subconscious Power
by Maxwell Maltz, M.D., F.I.C.S.

Contents:
1. The Self Image: Your Key to a Better Life 2. Discovering the Success Mechanism within You 3. Imagination—The First Key to Your Success Mechanism 4. Dehypnotize Yourself from False Beliefs 5. How to Utilize the Power of Rational Thinking 6. Relax and Let Your Success Mechanism Work for You 7. You Can Acquire the Habit of Happiness 8. Ingredients of the Success-Type Personality and How to Acquire Them 9. The Failure Mechanism: How to Make It Work For You Instead of Against You 10. How to Remove Emotional Scars, or How to Give Yourself an Emotional Face Lift 11. How to Unlock Your Real Personality 12. Do-It-Yourself Tranquilizers That Bring Peace of Mind 13. How to Turn a Crisis into a Creative Opportunity   **268 Pages... $2**

A PRACTICAL GUIDE TO SELF-HYPNOSIS
by Melvin Powers

Contents:
1. What You Should Know About Self-Hypnosis 2. What About the Dangers of Hypnosis? 3. Is Hypnosis the Answer? 4. How Does Self-Hypnosis Work? 5. How to Arouse Yourself From the Self-Hypnotic State 6. How to Attain Self-Hypnosis 7. Deepening the Self-Hypnotic State 8. What You Should Know About Becoming an Excellent Subject 9. Techniques for Reaching the Somnambulistic State 10. A New Approach to Self-Hypnosis When All Else Fails 11. Psychological Aids and Their Function 12. The Nature of Hypnosis   **120 Pages... $2**

A GUIDE TO RATIONAL LIVING

Contents: *by Albert Ellis, Ph.D. & Robert A. Harper, Ph.D.*

1. How Far Can You Go With Self-Analysis? 2. You Feel as You Think 3. Feeling Well by Thinking Straight 4. What Your Feelings Really Are 5. Thinking Yourself Out of Emotional Disturbances 6. Recognizing and Attacking Neurotic Behavior 7. Overcoming the Influences of the Past 8. How Reasonable is Reason? 9. The Art of Never Being Desperately Unhappy 10. Tackling Dire Needs for Approval 11. Eradicating Dire Fears of Failure 12. How to Stop Blaming and Start Living 13. How to Be Happy Though Frustrated 14. Controlling Your Own Destiny 15. Conquering Anxiety 16. Conquering Self-discipline 17. Rewriting Your Personal History 18. Accepting Reality 19. Overcoming Inertia and Becoming Creatively Absorbed   **208 Pages... $2**

A GUIDE TO SUCCESSFUL MARRIAGE
by Albert Ellis, Ph.D. & Robert A. Harper, Ph.D.
Contents:
1. Modern Marriage: Hotbed of Neurosis 2. Factors Causing Marital Disturbance 3. Gauging Marital Compatibility 4. Problem Solving in Marriage 5. Can We Be Intelligent About Marriage? 6. Love or Infatuation? 7. To Marry or Not To Marry 8. Sexual Preparation for Marriage 9. Impotence in the Male 10. Frigidity in the Female 11. Sex "Excess" 12. Controlling Sex Impulses 13. Non-monogamous Desires 14. Communication in Marriage 15. Children 16. In-laws 17. Marital Incompatibility Versus Neurosis 18. Divorce 19. Succeeding in Marriage 20. Selected Readings   **304 Pages... $2**

HOW YOU CAN HAVE CONFIDENCE & POWER

Contents: *by Les Giblin*

1. Your Key to Success and Happiness 2. How to Use the Basic Secret for Influencing Others 3. How to Cash in on Your Hidden Assets 4. How to Control the Actions & Attitudes of Others 5. How You Can Create a Good Impression on Other People 6. Techniques for Making & Keeping Friends 7. How to Use Three Big Secrets for Attracting People 8. How to Make the Other Person Feel Friendly—Instantly 9. How You Can Develop Skill in Using Words 10. The Technique of "White Magic" 11. How to Get Others to See Things Your Way—Quickly 12. A Simple, Effective Plan of Action That Will Bring You Success and Happiness.   **180 Pages... $2**

The books listed above can be obtained from your book dealer or directly from Wilshire Book Company. When ordering, please remit 15c per book postage. Send for our free 224 page illustrated catalog of self-improvement books.

Wilshire Book Company
12015 Sherman Road, No. Hollywood, California 91605